Yoga

The Best Guide to Yoga Practice, Calm Your Mind
and Improve Your Spirit

(Yoga Poses and Postures for Effective Weight
Loss, Restorative Yoga and Natural Self-healing)

Mark Lasater

Published by Rob Miles

Mark Lasater

All Rights Reserved

Yoga: The Best Guide to Yoga Practice, Calm Your Mind and Improve Your Spirit (Yoga Poses and Postures for Effective Weight Loss, Restorative Yoga and Natural Self-healing)

ISBN 978-1-989990-56-8

Legal & Disclaimer

The information contained in this book is not designed to replace or take the place of any form of medicine or professional medical advice. The information in this book has been provided for educational and entertainment purposes only.

The information contained in this book has been compiled from sources deemed reliable, and it is accurate to the best of the Author's knowledge; however, the Author cannot guarantee its accuracy and validity and cannot be held liable for any errors or omissions. Changes are periodically made to this book. You must consult your doctor or get professional medical advice before using any of the suggested remedies, techniques, or information in this book.

Table of Contents

Introduction

This book contains proven steps and strategies on how to understand the important concepts of yoga–mudras and asanas. This gives you a guide on how to begin yoga practices and what you need to know when you are only beginning to learn about yoga.

This makes it easier for you to understand the complex concepts of yoga. You can practice yoga no matter how old you are. This book contains a step-by-step guide on the right poses that you can easily follow. It offers tips and advices about what you need to know to make your yoga practice safe and effective.

Thanks again for downloading this book, I hope you enjoy it!

Chapter 1: The Fundamentals Of Asana

The direct translation of Asana, a Sanskrit term, describes a seat. It is a strange label until one realizes that a seat is not necessarily a chair. The seat referenced here is the balanced position that does not require any activation of forces to remain static. When one is seated correctly, the body will be able to remain in that position for long periods without having to move, realign, or stretch. Picture the term Asana as a posture that invokes balance.

When you see it this way, what flows naturally from that perspective is the compendium of physical postures and practices that serve to assuage the effects of imbalance. A key aspect of Asana is the combined consequence found in breathing and walking. Proper breathing techniques relax the muscles, reduce the acidity of the tissues and blood, and provide clarity to the mind.

The lifestyles that we face today differ a great deal compared to centuries past. Our body does not have the opportunity to realign itself naturally in the activities that we undertake the way it used to through various activities endemic to the lifestyle of the ancients. Breathing and walking – the two most important things to the human body are rarely done, and if done, are insufficient or incorrect.

This is where Asana comes in. Asana is not just about striking a pose. It's also about breathing correctly, hydrating adequately and learning to invoke calm. Look at it as stillness, motion, breathing, and hydration as the different aspects of this first limb of Yoga.

Stillness is to motion, as silence is to sound, and darkness is to light. We are typically taught to believe that stillness and silence are the absence of movement and sound. However, Yoga practitioners come to realize that stillness and silence are, in effect, vessels that hold motion and sound, just as darkness holds the light. By embracing the ability to identify and mimic stillness we are increasing our state of consciousness, not turning it off.

In parallel to stillness holding motion, silence holding sound, and darkness holding light, peace holds chaos. When we take the body from movement to stillness and sound to silence, we slowly transcend into other areas, especially the one that makes the most difference – from chaos to peace.

Posture

There are two aspects of any posture to be noted. Motion and stillness. Imagine a Yoga session where a person assumes a particular pose. It is most often misunderstood that the pose is the objective. The truth is that the pose is only half the story. The benefit is gained during the motion that gets the body into that pose, as well as when the body uncoils from that pose. This is the underlying reason that the method one uses to get to the pose is equally, if not more, important than the pose itself.

When attending Yoga classes, pay attention to the motion – the technique of getting to the pose, and how one uncoils from the pose. It is not sufficient to look at the image of the pose and find your way to it. This is the reason instructors are needed to guide the novice in striking the right pose and doing the right move.

The pose must also be balanced on the proper stance. The proper stance sets up the base of the posture. How a part of your body rests on the mat is important in keeping the forces in your body balanced. It is like standing on a flat surface versus on an incline. The posture you assume on an incline would require more energy and strain to stand erect than standing on a horizontal surface.

Once the posture is achieved, observe the alignment of your body. You should be able to lock everything in place – without applying tension to the muscles and yet remain in that position without trouble. If you get tired in a certain pose, it probably means that there is a build-up of acid in a certain muscle group. Acid build-up means that the posture is incorrectly struck and is unnatural.

There are two possible reasons for this unnatural state. Either the technique to get to the pose, or the pose itself is wrong. Or, the muscle groups which are affected by that pose are not properly stretched and out of balance. To overcome this, you have to get an instructor to advise on your pose, or you have to stretch the muscle groups that are not cooperating.

Breathing

Breathing is central to Yoga. To be able to gain the most benefit, proper breathing should be addressed early. Breathing happens in waves. It should not be shallow or rapid. Breathing happens in waves with shorter amplitude, punctuated by a wave of large amplitude. The frequency of breathing should be measured, and the lungs must be used to the fullest. Shallow breathing increases toxicity in the body, that we become used to over time. It also reduces the efficacy of the metabolic system and diminishes the full power of the mind. Most people only use half the volume of their lungs because of poor posture.

To breath correctly, imagine a balloon in your chest and think of a posture that does two things. First, open the chest area to allow that balloon within to expand, Second find the posture that balances the weight of your head and back without having to use any of your muscles to support it. Once you get there, you can let all your muscles gradually relax. Your diaphragm will do the rest.

Hydration

Everything in Yoga always comes back to the balance of still versus movement. Just as you saw in posture, hydration is not just about how much you drink, it's also about how much you expel. Water is the main component of your body. It is a part of all of you. From the structure of our brain to the content of your skin, water is the essential component that gives us life. More than that, it is also the moment of water that allows the human body to regulate heat, remove toxins, and lubricate various components of the body.

In Yoga, hydration is not just about drinking two liters of water a day, it is also about proper urination and perspiration habits. Yoga seeks to keep the body in balance and the materials that we are subjected to these days strain that balance. In the case of water, Yoga understands, and promotes, the need to have water move through the system frequently rather than store the water indefinitely.

We are not camels. We do not need to store large amounts of water. Our design requires water to enter and exit frequently. Merely drinking and waiting to empty the bladder is insufficient. Water needs to also move through evaporation from the lungs and nasal passages, it needs to exit through the skin. Expelling water through perspiration and breathing must also be done via the movement of the Asanas.

Chapter 2: Yoga Mudras Types And Effective Practices

Types of mudras

The various types of mudras are as follows.

Gyan Mudra: The gyan mudra raises the level of the element vayu or air in the body. This mudra is done by joining together the tip of the thumb and the index finger. Read More.

Prana Mudra: The pran mudra helps in increasing vitality and in the activation of the root chakrar To perform this mudra, you should keep the tips of your little finger, ring finger and thumb togethere

The middle and index finger should remain extendede Read Morer

Vayu Mudra: The meaning of vayu is 'wind', and this mudra is aimed specifically at getting rid of flatulencee It is said to produce immediate resultsu However, once the problem is relieved you should stop doing the posep Read MoreM

Prithvi Mudra: This mudra helps in activating the root chakrac The root chakra holds the elemental force of vital energye Some of the benefits of the prithvi mudra are increased energy, inner stability, and strengthening of the mind and bodyd Read Mored

Chin Mudra: The chin mudra is used in breathing exercises like Ujjayi Pranayama or in seated meditationd This mudra is effective for lower back pain, reducing stress, and for headachese Read Moree

Apaan Mudra: The apaan mudra is a very useful and important mudra that detoxifies the body and then energizes ite

Some of the benefits of apaan mudra are for constipation, anuria, and delayed child deliveryd Read More

Surya Mudra: The surya mudra helps decrease the earth element and increase the fire element in the body It is effective in regulating the metabolism and body temperature Read More>

Shunya Mudra: To perform this mudra, you should keep the thumb on the middle finger, while the remaining fingers are kept straight The benefits of this mudra include dealing with numbness in the body, vertigo, deafness, and earaches Read Morel

Linga Mudra: The linga mudra strengthens the immune system of the body and loosens the collected mucous in the bodyc This mudra is also effective for weight loss because of the generation of heatn Read Moret

Ganesha Mudra: The ganesha mudra symbolizes strength when faced with troublesa You should practice this mudra dailye It helps stimulate the metabolism and digestionl Read Morer

Mandala Mudra: The mandala mudra is practiced to symbolize the offering of the whole physical universe to the enlightened teachers and Buddha Although this pose is not created by the deities, it is employed extensively in the practice of ritual visualization called 'mandala offering'd Read Morer

Shankh Mudra: You can find this mudra in Hindu temples as symbolsn

This mudra is very effective for throat problemsv The clasping positioning of the fingers in this mudra simulates a conch shelli Read Mored

Rudra Mudra: To perform this mudra, you should keep the tips of the ring finger and index finger on top of the thumbs tipo The other fingers should be comfortably extended Read More-

Apan Vayu Mudra: This mudra is used in heart attacks as first aidh Regular practice of this mudra can help strengthen the heart Read Morev

Surahi Mudra: To perform this mudra, you should join the little fingers of both hands togethern The middle finger and forefinger should also be joined togethero Keep the thumbs freeg Read Morer

Surabhi Mudra: You can perform this mudra thrice a day for 15 minutesr This mudra is effective in dealing with rheumatic inflammation and helps increase intellectn Read Moreu

Hakini Mudra: This mudra helps improve coordination between the left and right hemispheres of the braind You can practice this mudra at anytime and anyplacei

Bronchial and Asthma Mudra: These mudras are effective for respiratory conditionsc You can practice them for a few minutes consecutively, till the breathing calms downy

Back Mudra: This mudra is very effective for dealing with backachee You can practice this mudra with both handsc

Kundalini Mudra: This mudra helps awaken the sexual force and unifies the feminine and masculinei You can practice this mudra thrice a day for 15 minutesu

Khechari Mudra: Practicing this mudra enables the release of neurotransmitters like dopamine This helps bring about a state of well being and calmnesss

Yoni Mudra: This mudra is used to bring isolation to your senses and keep you from distractionss This can help you look inward with a calm and relaxed minda

Jnana Mudra: In this mudra, the hands with the palms facing up are kept on the knees in the seated positiont This mudra gives a spacious feeling and uplifts the mind and bodyn

Chapter 3: What Is Yoga?

The word 'yoga' is procured from the Sanskrit term (root) 'yuj' that signifies 'to unite',' to join' and 'to attach'. Yoga is defined as mental, spiritual and physical disciplines and practices that pioneered in ancient India. Its main objective is to earn imperishable and perdurable peace of mind to confront one's true and authentic self.' Union with the divine' or yoga has been extracted from yuj Samadhi meaning to concentrate and yujir yoga meaning to yoke; two roots. Yoga is associated with Buddhism, Jainism and Hinduism. It is critical part of Hindu, Tibetan Buddhist philosophy and Varjrayana. The pivotal aspiration of yoga is liberation (moksha). Yoga has been often described as the pioneer and triumph consequence of Globalization. Western world celebrated Hatha yoga, a form of yoga celebrated as it become admirable as a system of physical exercise'. Swami Vivekanand and certain Gurus of India announced Yoga to the west. It is an interesting fact that, at present, more people practice yoga in West than in India. Yoga is 5,000 years old. Thoreau was the first Yogi preaching in America.

A person who follows, yoga philosophy and yoga with a sense of commitment and devotion is called a 'yogi' (male or female), while yogini refers to female who dedicate themselves to yoga and its philosophy. Yoga is appraised as an epitome of spirituality. Its supreme aim is cessation and abandonment of fluctuation and instability of human mind. Yoga is quite more than mastering poses and postures and enhancing strength and flexibility. The traditional purpose of Yoga has always been able to bring profound and deep transformation in the person through the transcendence of the ego.

The origin of Yoga is still unresolved and dubious. Its initial inceptions and inauguration is often linked with Indus Valley Civilization, in Vedic period including, the Upanisadas, Bhagavat Gita,

17

Mahabarata, Early Buddhism, Jainism, and Yoga Sutras of Patanjali and in the Middle-Ages, including the Bhakti Movement, Tantra and Sikhism. Patanjali is acknowledged as the "father of Yoga'. He inscribed scriptures, popular as Yoga Sutras and series of crucial verses.

Yoga has eight fundamental and vital limbs or branches. These are sets of philosophical and lifestyle guidelines that includes:

Yama, referred as five abstentions namely, truth, celibacy, non-violence, non-possessiveness and non-stealing

Niyama it is a blend of five observances that includes, austerity, contentment, purity, surrender to God and approaching God through Vedic scriptures

Asana depicts 'seat' for meditation

Pranayam denotes control of life force through suspending breath

Pratyhara refers to disengagement of sense organs from the superficial world.

Dharana symbolizes concentration or engrossment

Dhyana indicates 'meditation'

Samadhi represents 'liberation' of the soul.

The calm steadiness of the sense is called peace. Then one should become watchful, because yoga comes and goes'-Katha Upanishad Yoga is often co-related with religion but it's erroneous to scrutinize it with religion. Instead it is an expression of spirituality. It is a classical form of meditation that synchronizes our mind, body, breath and soul by establishing a sense of awareness. It has enormous physical and psychological benefits. The eight chakras of our body namely Anahata, Bindu, Mooladhara, Ajna, Sashara, Vishuddhi, Manipura and Swadhisthana are purified and refined by yoga practices by balancing our Bandhans or energy locks. However, some yogis and yoginis circumvent yoga practices on New and Full moon days as the moon affects our emotions. New Moons are 'vacant, empty and clear, hence, they signifies reconstruction of our projects, commitments, relationships and ideas. The Full Moon alters our emotions, agreements, relationships and projects as the moon influences the water within us, hence, averting a few from yoga for a day (it is infrequent though).

Yoga has certainly many enlightening facts. Its powerful breathing system aids in flexibility. Flexibility is associated more with the mind than with the body. Yoga, being a breathing practice, preaches the Lungs as the most vital and crucial organ of the body. All the yoga practices are closely interwoven to slow the rhythm and expanding the capacity of breaths for longevity and healthy life. 'For breath is life, and if you breath well you will live long on earth'-a Sanskrit Proverb. Our breath reveals and signifies our mood. By altering breath, we can improve and modify our moods. Hence, it's good for a healthy and peaceful mind.

As Sharon Gannon said that 'You cannot do yoga. Yoga is your natural state'. What you can do are yoga exercises which may reveal to you where you are resisting your natural state. As yoga is an ancient concept of physical discipline but it's always about physiological and spiritual well-being. Fundamentally, all yoga types and styles strive to deliver the same outcome, the unification of mind, body, spirit and soul. They may vary, so long as philosophy is concerned. There are ten disciplines of yoga but Kundalini Yoga, Astanga Yoga and Hatha Yoga are the most common yet popular disciplines.

Ashtanga Yoga. It is modern day version of classical Indian Yoga. It incorporates the unifying and integrated discipline of the eight limbs. Power Yoga and Vinyasa yoga are derived from Astanga Yoga.

Hatha Yoga. It is constructed on pranayams (breathing techniques or breathe control) and asanas (postures or physical activity).

Kundalini Yoga. Infleunced by the Tantra and Shakta schools of Hinduism it is based on deriving the Kundalani Energy (kundalini shakti) by incorporating meditation, asanas, chanting mantras and pranayam.

Yoga is a science of mental discipline and self-culture. It brings wisdom, nobility and sagacity in human beings. Yoga is for everyone, mindless their sex, age, caste, creed and even religion. It is benevolent and beneficial and almost anyone can reap its rewards. It is fallacious that it's a kind of mental and physical acrobatics. Enjoy the gift of Yoga with its tremendous wealth and vastness. Anyone can resolve psychological, mental, physical and emotional issues with yoga and heal your mind, body and soul. It is an inexpensive and exciting form that would lead your way to overall wellness.

Chapter 4: The Different Types Of Yoga

As with anything in life, one thing does not suit everyone; the great thing about yoga however, is that there is a type which will suit you, you just need to know about the different ones, and the ways to adapt them to your situation and circumstances.

When searching for a yoga class, you will probably find the more mainstream types of yoga come up more frequently, but if you really do want to try a more obscure or rare type of yoga, you will find it but probably in a larger city, for example. Of course, you can teach yourself too, and we'll go over the pros and cons of classes vs home teaching a little later in the book.

For now, let's explore the different types of yoga you can try.

Anusara yoga

We're going to start alphabetically here, so obviously first up we have Anusara. This is one of the newer versions of yoga, a

24

discipline which is always developing and adapting to our lifestyles and needs. Anusara is based around the fact that everyone is filled with good, and the poses used in this type of yoga is designed to allow you to open up your heart chakra.

Anusara is quite a physical workout, but it can also be quite mentally tiring too, so perhaps not the best idea to begin with this type of yoga if you are totally new to the discipline. Having said that, if you are struggling with your levels of self-esteem or self-confidence and your fitness levels are reasonably good, you can certainly give this type of yoga a try.

Ashtanga yoga

You may have heard about ashtanga yoga in the press or magazines, as this is a particular favorite amongst celebrities currently. Those with a good standard of physical strength and stamina can give this one a go, because ashtanga is certainly a work out and a half!

Each class is made up of the same series of poses, which you move from and to using your breath to help the sequence move smoothly and easily.

Bikram yoga

Again, this is another celebrity favourite, and you've probably heard Madonna talking about how great this type of yoga is for your mind and body. Again, this is a very demanding type, and it is actually done in a heated room – you will certainly sweat!

Each class is made up of 26 different poses and each one is done in the same order for each class, so you're not going to get any surprises.

Hatha yoga

If you're looking for a pretty general form of yoga to give a try first of all, then hatha is for you; this is also the most common form of yoga you'll find in classes in sports centres and hotels/spas etc. This is a very low impact form of yoga, which is ideal for beginners or those with mobility or flexibility problems. By the end of the class you can expect to feel quite relaxed and chilled out, but you will certainly be getting a gentle and subtle work out at the same time, probably without even realizing it.

Hatha classes are made up of the most basic yoga poses, which are moved through in smooth sequences by using breath.

Iyengar yoga

If you have previous injury which impairs your mobility to a degree or you have problems holding poses due to balance issues, iyengar yoga is a good one for you to try. This type of yoga incorporates props, such as chairs or bolsters, into the sequence of poses, to give you a support as you move from one to another.

Despite that description, iyengar is quite challenging in terms of fitness and mental fatigue, because in order to follow the sequence and do them right (this is very important in iyengar yoga) you really need to concentrate. You will also find that your yoga teacher is going to be watching your posture within the poses and how you move from one to the other very carefully, and will correct you if need be.

Vinyasa yoga

Vinyasa yoga is a good source of middle ground because it gives you a high quality work out, whilst not being too demanding at the same time; this is a good one to try if you're of an intermediate level.

Vinyasa yoga classes don't tend to have much in the way of pauses in them, and you will be moving for much of the time. There are a series of poses which you will work through, using your breath as an aid, without stopping between them.

Restorative yoga

This is the most laid-back type of yoga there is, and it is idea for anyone who is trying to come back from a depressive episode, or anyone who suffers from stress and anxiety. Restorative yoga focuses on the mind and wellbeing in that department, using relaxation techniques and simple poses to get the job done. You're not going to get the most physical workout from a restorative yoga class, but you will get a mood boost, and perhaps that is more important in some cases.

You don't have to stick to just one type of yoga, because it's perfectly acceptable to try out a few, before you find the best one for you, or maybe the best ones for you. As you become more proficient and flexible, you can move up in ability level, and you can try other, more demanding yoga classes, such as bikram, for example.

How to Find the Right Type of Yoga For You

If you have looked at our various described types of yoga and identified one or more types you want to try, here is how to find a class:

- Check local newspaper listings

- Enquire at your local sports club

- Check out large hotels, e.g. those with a fitness centre or spa, for example

- Look at social media groups, e.g. yoga groups on Facebook

- Check to see if any small public places have independent classes running, e.g. village halls, schools, church halls, etc

- Google further afield if you really want to try a specific type of yoga and you're unable to find in your local area

- Check out yoga retreats, you could even head overseas to enjoy a yoga holiday!

Finding a yoga class to suit you isn't difficult for most of the common types of yoga, and bikram yoga is one of the most popular at the moment – this is something you will find on the program of most large spots clubs these days, simply because it's so in fashion at the moment. The key is simply to search around carefully, and perhaps try a couple of different types of yoga before deciding on the one that suits you best.

Yoga is For Everyone, How to Adapt it to Your Needs

Everyone has specific needs, e.g. perhaps you have a chronic injury which is long-standing and requires you to adapt the way you move, perhaps you're pregnant, perhaps you have a risk of back injury from time to time, or perhaps you simply have limited flexibility or mobility, perhaps due to age. The important thing to realize here is that yoga is for everyone, and it's simply a case of adapting your practice to suit your needs.

We should also point out there that just because you don't think you're getting the biggest cardio workout from a yoga class, this doesn't mean that you're not! Yoga is subtly very effective, and you will actually sweat much more than you might realize! If you're using yoga as part of a weight management program, you may be very surprised at the effect it has on your efforts!

A good quality yoga teacher will be able to give you advice on this, and will also be able to keep an eye on any part of the class which is not suitable for you, simply by informing you of this (in a confidential way, so none of the class hears), and will also give you an alternative pose to do, so you don't miss out on any part of the work out. Of course, if you do have any health issues or injuries, you should follow these two golden rules:

• Talk to your doctor before you begin, to check your suitability

• Talk to your yoga teacher, to make them aware of any adapted poses you may need during the class

If you tick these two boxes, there's no reason why you can't enjoy and benefit from yoga, just like everyone else.

Now we've covered the basics of yoga, and we know about the different types, let's talk about the major health benefits you can expect to receive.

Chapter 5: Yoga For Weight Loss

Before we get into using yoga to lose weight it is important for you to understand that yoga is not going to work any miracles in your life. Just like any other way of losing weight, you have to focus on all of the areas of your life.

Yoga is just like any other exercise when it comes to losing weight. Yes, it is going to strengthen your body. Yes, it is going to give you more energy. Yes, it is going to burn more calories and boost your metabolism, but if you want to lose weight you have to focus on other areas as well.

Using yoga to lose weight is great because the exercises are not fast paced. This means that if you have never exercised before you will be strengthening your muscles, but you are going to have to focus on your diet and hydration as well.

There is also no one size fits all technique to losing weight, but there are techniques that anyone can use to make it easier. The first thing that you need to focus on is what you are putting into your body. Many people forget this aspect because they think since they are exercising they should be losing weight, but if you are not giving your body the proper fuel, your body is not going to be able to function properly. This means that your body is not going to be able to burn fat properly.

Focus on eating natural whole foods, plant based meals and reducing the amount of meat that you eat. Cut back on refined sugars and processed foods if you want to see the biggest results. You also want to focus on hydration. Our bodies are made up of more than 70 percent water and if you are not giving your body the water that it needs you cannot expect it to function properly or burn fat properly. Often times people are amazed at how much weight they lose when they begin drinking enough water. This is because if you are not drinking enough water your body will hold on to fat because it is easier to store fat than it is to burn it this way the body is able to hold on to the water that it does have.

In order to lose weight with yoga you will need to follow the following routine at least 3 times each week and hold each position for at least 3 breaths and up to 5 breaths unless stated otherwise.

Crescent - This exercise helps to firm the abs, hips as well as the thighs.

Begin by standing with your feet together, toes pointed forward and your arms at your sides. Begin inhaling and as you do raise your arms over your head reaching your fingertips toward the ceiling. Exhale and as you do bend forward at the hip, placing your hands on the floor. Inhale again and as you exhale you will move your right foot back one step, bending your left knee until you are in a lunge position. Inhale again raising your arms overhead and looking at the ceiling. Hold this position for three to five breaths and return to the beginning position. Repeat, alternating which foot you step back with each time.

Willow Position - This helps to firm the oblique muscles.

Begin this exercise by standing with your feet together and your arms at your sides. Raise the left leg, placing the sole of your left foot against the inside of your right thigh. Stretch your arms out in front of you bringing your palms together in front of your chest and hold for two breaths. When you inhale for the third time, raise your arms extending your fingertips as if you are trying to reach the ceiling. When you exhale you will bend your torso left. Straighten as you inhale. Repeat this three to five times, keeping the left foot pressed into the right thigh. Return to the starting position and switch sides.

Rocking the Boat - This Firms that abs and strengthens the back.

Begin this pose by sitting on the floor with your knees bent, feet flat on the floor and your hands resting on your thighs. Keeping your torso straight, as well as your head and neck you will lean back 45 degrees. Raise your feet and calves, keeping them parallel to the floor and your toes should be pointed. As you inhale you will stretch your arms and legs out forming a V with your body and using your arms to balance yourself. Exhale then as you inhale again lower your torso and your legs about 3 inches so that you are creating a wider V shape. Exhale and raise your torso and legs back up. Repeat this three to five times.

Hover Position - This will firm the shoulders, arms, abs and strengthen the back.

To begin this position place yourself in the push-up position with your arms straight, toes bent and hands below your shoulders ensuring that your body is in line from one end to the other. As you exhale, lower your chest toward the floor, bending your elbows so that the top of your arm is parallel with your body, keeping them close to your sides. Hold yourself in position just a few inches above the floor for three to five breaths.

The Chair Position - This helps to firm the butt and thighs.

Begin by standing with your feet together, toes pointing forward and your arms at your sides. Inhale deeply and raise your arms over your head. Your palms should be facing each other. Exhale and move into sitting position (about 45 degrees) it should look as if you are getting ready to sit down. Hold this position for three to five breaths. Straighten your legs, lower your arms and repeat.

Of course, doing these yoga exercises is going to help you lose weight, but you need to remember to focus on the other areas of your life as well. Yoga is considered strength training and stretching so you should consider adding in an aerobic exercise on the days that you do not do yoga. Do not forget how important diet and hydration is when it comes to losing weight as well.

Chapter 6: Yoga Etiquette That You Need To Know

Good manners may seem really hard to come by especially in our over-worked, stressed out community. We may all use some yoga now more than ever. Along with its promise for a healthier well-being and deep inner peace, it is no surprise that the ancient practice of yoga continues to be very popular in the Western countries. A recent yoga journal reported that about 14 million individuals in the United States alone have practiced some form of yoga in 2010. With the ever growing of yogis, occasional ruffled feathers may tend to be unavoidable. Below are some yoga etiquettes to observe when attending yoga classes:

Be quiet please. This may seem like a no-brainer. Before attending a yoga class, make sure to turn off your cell phone. It will also be a very bad idea to make a loud entrance or exit in yoga class. Just a little reminder just like in the movie theater before the show starts, please be quiet or make as little noise as possible while you get settled for your yoga class.

If you show up late, tiptoe in class

Showing up late in yoga class in very inevitable, but it would be very polite to wait until everybody is finished with their starting meditation and be as quiet as a mice as not to interrupt with the peace.

During the Dharma talk, be respectful by making eye contact with your yoga instructor

Eye contact is very much a strong manifestation of respect. When your instructor is talking about how the practice of yoga have modified their life or sharing certain traditional philosophy teachings; give your undivided, full attention. Even if you do not like the manner your instructor is providing the material, try your very best to keep concentrated. So instead of closing your eyes or lying down, be attentive. You may just discover something new from your yoga instructor.

Follow what your instructor is teaching and don't try adding your own "flair"

It is very disrespectful when you try to do your own thing. Your yoga instructor places a great deal of effort and time to prepare for the class and do it with great purpose. Your yoga instructor may most likely attended several workshops, read books on yoga and practice regularly to perfect their craft. There is something great about letting yourself to be led and just experience what your instructor has to offer. If there is certain yoga pose that you feel you can't live without, you are always free to do it when your yoga class is over.

Attending a yoga class is a "work in""and not a "work out

Whenever you take a group exercise session, bike, run or lift weights, you work up a sweat and experience a good workout. Yoga on the other hand, is a traditional system for overall well-being where participants learn to widen the conscious mind deeper into the subconscious mind. The ultimate goal is to learn to live in union with other people and with nature. The principle of yoga is a shift to the inner-most self and a technique to see the divine and true nature. Therefore, it is best to regard yoga as a "work in".

Don't take over the skylight

Perhaps you have your favorite spot in the yoga studio – by the windy window, beneath the skylight and right in front of the yoga instructor, however be adaptable. A morning yoga class on a Saturday may get quite jam packed, and you do not wish to be that person who refuses to move his/her mat a few inches to the right since it will ruin the view.

Do not walk across other yogis' mats

To look for a spot to roll you matt out, keep from touching other's mat. No one likes another person's sweaty feet to be touching their stuff.

Do not laugh

Don't laugh at the old man wearing an American flag in the front row, your friend or even at yourself. However, you should feel free to smile every now and then. Yogis should also know how to have fun.

Do not be a human sprinkler

Yoga practice can really get you sweaty, so take a towel with you during every class. Dripping sweat all over the other person's mat next to you is sort of like peeing on another person's carpet. Angry glares are absolutely to take place.

Do not rush out of class

If you rush out of class, you may step on innocent hands or knock over water bottles during savasana. Relax, you just spent all that time doing all that yoga poses.

Chapter 7: Introductory Exercises

When you are starting to do yoga, you have to remember that it's very much like any other activity of this nature. You can't go straight into doing exercises without first preparing yourself. This includes stretching exercises that allow you to limber up and get ready for your yoga session. In this chapter, we deal with warming up exercises – from which you will be able to move on to more complex exercises.

Breathing

In many exercises in yoga, the breathing in and out goes with the actions that you take. Thus, it's important to learn to breathe in the most efficient way. If you can take a position on your mat and make sure that your back is straight, this will help the efficiency of the breathing. When you breathe in, count to seven and make sure that you breathe in through the nose. Hold the breath for a moment and then breathe out through the nose. Concentrate on your breathing and be aware of the important part this has in yoga. If you have adopted the habit of breathing through your mouth, you do need to concentrate on nasal breathing as this is much more effective.

Exercises to warm up

Leg exercise

Stand on your yoga mat and bend your leg back as far as you can from the knee. Hold onto the leg because this helps you to work the muscles in the leg. Pull the leg in toward your bottom and at the same time push the leg firmly against your hand. What this does is work all the muscles in your leg. During this exercise, keep your back straight and remember to point the knee down toward the ground. This will help you with leg strengthening but it will also help you considerably with your posture. Keep in this position for a short while, breathe out and release the leg standing on both feet once again. Then work on the other leg.

This time do the same thing again with the first leg and when you hold your leg, hold it with both hands and make sure that you work your shoulders back as far as they will go. This really does reinforce standing straight and is useful for the shoulders and the legs, as well as being a great warm up exercise for beginners.

Asanas

As you begin your yoga experience, you need to understand that the movements that you do during the course of a yoga session are called Asanas. Some of these have names that you will learn very quickly. As a beginner, the warm up exercises below are suggested to help you to get your body ready for more complex yoga. It's important to remember that your body is not accustomed to this kind of exercise and you should therefore take your initial practice only as far as the body is comfortable with.

Sitting position

You may have seen people curling their legs into what looks like a very uncomfortable pose to do yoga. Fortunately for you, you don't have to do this at the beginning of your yoga experience. Sit on your mat with your back straight. Bend your legs and find a position that is comfortable where your ankles cross. It helps to use your yoga cushion because this props up the bottom and allows you to fold your legs in front of you more easily. This is also great for yoga meditation.

Place your hands onto your knees and while you do this remember that you need to feel as tall as you can so think through the movement of your body as you "think big" and stretch your back.

Neck exercises

Keeping your back as straight as it was at the beginning, move your head over to the right hand side and breathe in as you do so, breathe out and feel the air coursing through your body as you keep your head in this position. Keep your head there for several moments and then as you breathe out, move your head back to the central position. Although you may think that this will have little effect on losing weight or balancing your body, you'd actually be quite wrong. Yoga uses all of the areas of the body and the more efficient they get at movement and the more balanced the chakras, the more able your body is to function to an optimal level. Now, move the head to the other side and do the same thing.

Inhale and as you do so, move your head so that you are looking over your left shoulder, keep it there for a moment, and remember on your exhale, move it back to center. Do this for both sides. This helps to free up the neck of stiffness and should only be practiced within the level of your own comfort. Do not force it.

Body stretching

From the original seated position, it's time to stretch your body, so it's important to place your hands onto the mat, rather than onto your knees. From this position breathe in and as you do so, lift one arm as far over your head as you can. As you exhale slide the hand that is on the mat over as far as you can and take the other hand over the head as far as you are able without hurting yourself at all. The idea of this exercise is to stretch the side of body where the arm is in the air. Keep this position for a few moments and the next time that you breathe in, go back to center again, placing your hand on the mat beside you where you began. This needs doing on both sides so that you have stretched your body sufficiently. Remain within your comfort zone at all times and do not push yourself too far too quickly.

The waist

I love this exercise because it makes your body feel so balanced. Staying in the same seated position, place your right hand on your left knee and twist your body around from the waist. Remember the breathing. You breathe in as you move, you exhale and inhale as you keep that position then you exhale and move back to the original position. When you start doing this warm up exercise, you can actually hold the position for several breaths and then move back to the central position and repeat the exercise on the other side.

These are merely warm up exercises and in the next chapter, we will discuss the yoga poses more so that you can see how to do them and learn what benefits they have. Don't try to exercise too quickly and remember this isn't about sports. It's about feeling comfortable in the skin you're in, so there is no race. Take it slowly and move onto doing yoga poses when you are ready.

Chapter 8: How To Stretch Your Foot

For some of these stretches, it really does help to have something to prop your toes on. I like to use a yoga block, but a corner of a wall can work as well. If you prefer a yoga block, then you can often find one for less than $10. My favorite places to get yoga blocks are target or TJ Maxx but since yoga has become so popular, you can find them all over the place. You don't need to spend a lot of money on a yoga block. I've yet to find one that doesn't work well. However if you don't want to purchase a yoga block, then using the wall or something similar to a yoga block is just fine.

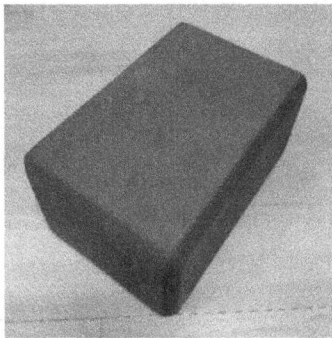

Yoga Block

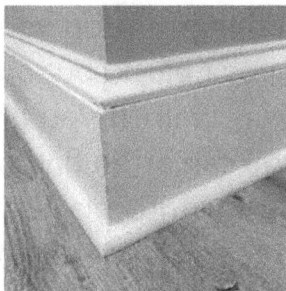

Corner of a wall

Toe Stretches

I use these toe stretches in yoga classes frequently, and my yoga students love it! I suggest that you practice your balance before you begin to stretch your toes. This will help illustrate to you just how much you can benefit from stretching out those feet.

Exercise: For this balance pose (from a standing position), simply lift up one foot. It doesn't have to be lifted up very high. Just lift your foot off of the floor. Then close your eyes. Notice your balance and when you're ready, switch sides and try it on the other foot. Once you've done that, then you are ready to move on to the stretches below.

There are 3 main versions of toe stretches that I like to do with my students. Try them all to see what works best for your own feet.

Stretch 1

For the first one, place all of your toes of your right foot on a block or wall and let the foot slide down the block. Hold this position for about a minute. If you've never stretched your foot, that minute might feel like a lifetime, but stay with it. It really doesn't take a long hold in order to begin to change your foot. A minute is plenty of time to begin to stretch that connective tissue in your foot.

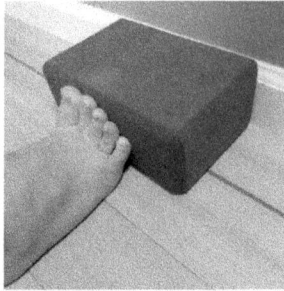

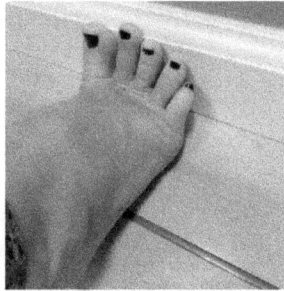

Stretch 2

For the second one, you'll go over to the right corner of the same block (or find a position on a wall where you can do this). Place your big toe on the block and let the other four toes go down to the floor. Again, you only need to hold this about a minute. That minute may seem like a short time, but it's enough to begin to have healthier feet.

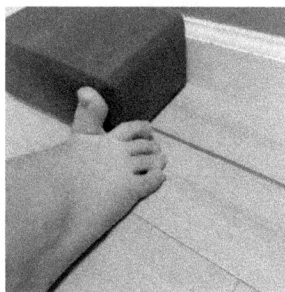

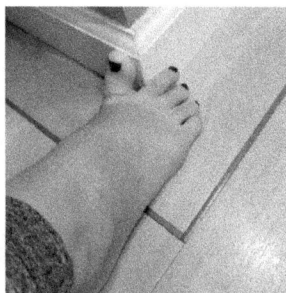

Stretch 3

For the third one, go over to the left corner of the block and place your four toes on the block and let the big toe go down to the floor. Now, I've found that with many people, the big toe won't easily go down to the floor. If that is happening for you, then you can use the other foot to encourage the toe down to the floor. Yes, I do mean to step on it and push it down, gently, of course. Again, hold for about a minute.

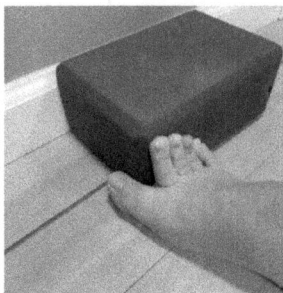

Now, after you have completed these toes

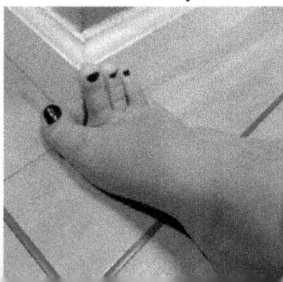

stretches on the right foot, pause to place both feet flat on the floor. Notice the difference in those feet. I always feel like my foot is much more awake after doing these stretches, and it's very obvious when I have done one foot and not the other one yet. After comparing your feet, repeat the above 3 stretches for your left foot. You'll do all the toes, move to the left corner of the block and have the big toe up and the other toes down, and then move to the right corner of the block so that the four toes are on the block and the big toe is down on the floor.

Exercise: Now that you've stretched both feet, go back to that balance pose that I had you do first. Try it on both sides. Notice your balance. Has it improved?

For the majority of people that I have worked with in a yoga class, the answer to whether your balance is better is a definite yes. Your feet can function so much better just by adding in some simple stretches. It will take you maybe 10 minutes to do all of these stretches as well as the balance pose before and after the stretches. What would it be like to have your feet feel better? Is it worth 10 minutes a couple of times a week to change your feet?

I think that investing time in your feet to help them feel better is a smart investment, and you will too once you begin to take more care of your feet. These simple stretches are the basis of what I've given to countless people in my yoga classes over the years. This is what has had so many people come back to me weeks or even months later and make a point of saying how much better their feet feel. Occasionally, I'll give them a few other pointers on things that they can do for their feet. However, the majority of people that I teach get just these stretches and walk away happier with their feet then they've been in a long time.

You can stop here and just do these few stretches and you'll begin to feel better. However, if you'd like to take your foot health even further, then read on to get some more tips and ideas for the healthiest feet that you've had in a long time.

Chapter 9

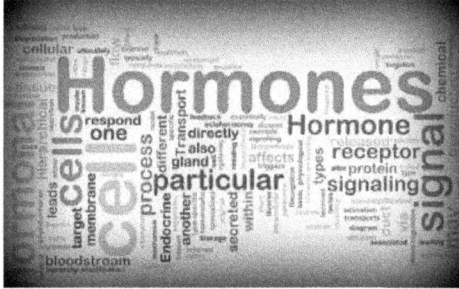

The endocrine system secretes hormones directly into the bloodstream and so the glands are known as ductless glands. The endocrine glands include:

Thepinealgland
Pituitarygland
Pancreas
Ovaries
Testes
Thyroid
Parathyroidgland
Hypothalamus
Adrenal glands

Some glands produce a single hormone and other glands produce two or more.

But let's take a more in-depth look at the function of the endocrine glands. **Pineal**-the function of this gland was obscured for a long time and is the last discovery in relation to the endocrine system. Once known as the 3rd eye, it produces melatonin and this helps to maintain the circadian rhythm and serves to regulate the reproductive hormones.

Pituitary-often known as the master gland, it influences most ductless glands within the body via its hormones.

The thyroid -this gland is important for the metabolism and it regulates the chemistry of the body's tissues. It's an important gland. It regulates the consumption of oxygen and the expulsion of carbon dioxide. When the gland is underactive, it can affect both physical and mental growth in children but in adults, the metabolic rate slows and so the side-effects are that the individual feels more lethargic, puts on weight and the mind will also slow down. When the thyroid gland is overactive, the opposite occurs. The individual may seem excited and even nervous in action and behaviour and weight loss is common. Pulse rate will also be rapid.

Parathyroid glands -these are two pairs of small oval glands which are embedded in the posterior surface of the thyroid. Under secretion will trigger the muscles to go into spasm, if over secretion occurs, the bones may soften. In addition, depression of the nervous system may also occur.

Thymus It is closely connected to the immune system and plays an important role in the development of T-lymphocytes or T cells. (An important type of white blood   cell).
 Adrenal glands– The secretion of the adrenal glands occur through anger or fear, also, as a result of starvation or asphyxia

The islets of Langerhans of the pancreas – concerned with the secretion of insulin. This lowers the concentration of glucose in the blood and facilitates transportation of glucose, along with potassium.

Ovaries– The internal female reproductive organs **Testes–** The internal male organ where testosterone is produced.
The nervous system
Divided into two parts, there is the central (Cerebrospinal) and autonomic system. The autonomic system is dependent on the cerebrospinal nervous system. The Cerebrospinal nervous system includes:

Thebrain
Thespinal-cord
The peripheral nerves

There are 31 pairs of nerves emerging from the spinal-cord and each of these nerves have 2 routes known as the anterior which carries the motor nerves and the posterior carrying sensory nerves. The motor nerves are responsible for carrying impulses to the muscles and so, for physical movement. The sensory nerves are responsible for sensory impulses and so send information along to the brain regarding sensation experienced.

The nerves are so named due to the section of the spine from which they emerge:

8pairs of cervical nerves
12 pairs of thoracic nerves
5 pairs of lumbar nerves
5 pairs of sacral nerves
1 pair of coccygeal nerves

There are also 12 pairs of cranial nerves, some are motor nerves, some are sensory.

Cranial nerves

Olfactory-the sensory nerve of smell
Optic-the sensory nerve of sight
Ocular motor-a motor nerve supplying most of the eye muscles
Trochlear-motor nerve to the external oblique eye muscle
Trigeminal -the largest of the cranial nerves. Both sensory and motor, it supplies most of the skin of the head and face, the teeth and the membranes of the

nose and mouth. Abducens -the motor nerves connected to the lateral rectus muscle of the eyeball Facial-both motor and sensory. It is mainly a motor nerve for muscles relating to the facial expressions and to the scalp. But it is sensory and connected to taste. Acoustic-the sensory nerve of hearing Glosso-Pharyngeal - a motor nerve to the muscle of the pharynx, secreto-motor re the parotid gland, and sensory for part of the tongue and the soft palate. It is the nerve of taste Vagus - a mixed nerves and it supplies the larynx, pharynx, lungs, heart, stomach, oesophagus and the liver Spinal accessoryalthough considered a motor nerve, it has two parts. One part accompanies the vagus, the other connects to the trapezius and sterno-mastoid muscles. Hypoglossal - motor nerve for the muscles of the tongue

Cranial nerves have numbers relative to its position and the numbers may be used instead of the above names. This is not relevant in terms of yoga but for awareness.

Self-Assessment Tasks

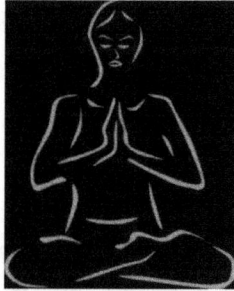

Task:

How many pairs of cranial nerves are there?

Task:

What is the pituitary gland often referred as?

Task:

State the two parts of the nervous system
Please note that these self-assessment tasks are to ensure your understanding of the information within each module. As

such, do not submit them for review with KEW Training Academy.

Chapter 10: Back Pain

Our modern, sedentary lifestyle has made back pain a fact of life. Slouching and sitting behind a desk all day make back pain so much worse. For those suffering from arthritis and osteoporosis, which often go hand in hand, treating back pain is absolutely necessary to living a quality, pain-free life.

The exercises in this section will help you reduce stress and tension that put even further strain on your back. They will also help you increase flexibility and build muscles that will protect and support your spine, and help prevent back pain in the future.

For those days when the pain is just too much to handle, this chapter also includes relaxing poses that will help you breathe through the pain.

Supported Bridge Pose

Sanskrit name: Setu Bandha Sarvangasana

Supported Bridge is one of the most calming poses in the yoga canon. It's a modification of traditional Bridge Pose, and a prep for Wheel Pose. Supported Bridge is the perfect pose for opening up the hips and back, which have taken a beating from hunching over a computer or desk all day. Adding a block or cushion allows your front hips and lower back to open in a way that's just too delicious. Add this into your routine at the end of the day to help you fall asleep or unwind after work.

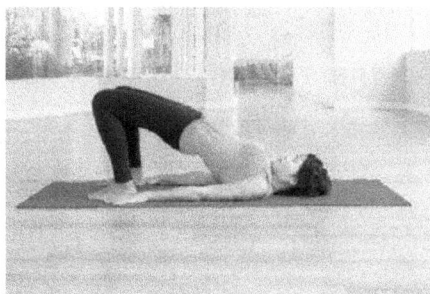

Instructions

Begin by reclining on your yoga mat.

Bring your feet flat on the ground and move them closer to your body, creating a bend in the knees.

Use your leg strength to lift your buttocks a few inches off of the ground. If needed, insert the block or rolled towel beneath your sacrum (lower back) and adjust until it is comfortable.

Breathe, and allow gravity to stretch your hips and lower back.

Props

This pose calls for a yoga block, rolled towel, or cushion. You can also use a towel or blanket under your head if your head hurts on the ground, but do not elevate your head enough to cause any strain in the neck.

Another option is to balance on a yoga bolster. Place the bolster vertically down your spine and relax.

Supine Twisting Posture

Sanskrit name: Jathara Parivartanasana

Supine Twist is a gentle pose that's perfect for beginners. It's also one of the poses that is deeply calming for the central nervous system, making it a great way to wind down at the end of the day.

This pose is very grounding because your entire body is touching the earth, so if you're feeling jittery or flighty, add this pose into your routine. Plus, it's a twist, which means it's detoxifying and can help with any digestive symptoms you may be suffering from thanks to autoimmune disease or painkillers.

When it comes to arthritis, you might hear some glorious back cracking when you enter this posture. This pose will create space in your back where before there was just tension. Basically, all parts of your body are connected to your spine – that's why back pain is so brutal. Aligning your spine and reducing tension in your lower back can go a long way to reducing chronic pain all over your body. As an added bonus, this pose will also bring a stretch and release to your shoulders, another body part often hit hard by arthritis.

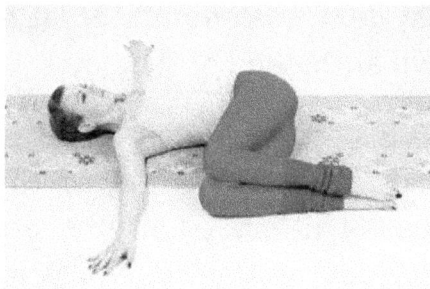

Instructions

Recline on your back on your yoga mat.

Bring your arms out wide into a T position.

Bring your knees to your face, and drape them over to the right side of your body. Turn your neck to look in the opposite direction and allow gravity to work on bringing your knees to the ground.

To maintain the stretch to your shoulders, make sure your shoulders remain flat on the ground.

Breathe, and remain in this posture as long as it is comfortable.

Props

This pose is simple and gentle, so it doesn't need many props. However, if your knees are sensitive, you can put a blanket beneath them.

If your hips are too tight for your knees to reach the floor, try placing a block beneath your knees.

Modifications

If you'd like to encourage more of a stretch, place your hand on the knee to gently push it downwards towards the floor.

Cobra Pose

Sanskrit name: Bhujangasana

Cobra Pose is a great transition pose during vinyasa. It serves to opens up the chest, shoulders, and back of the legs. Most importantly, it brings a stretch to your entire back, helping to reduce pain all over your body.

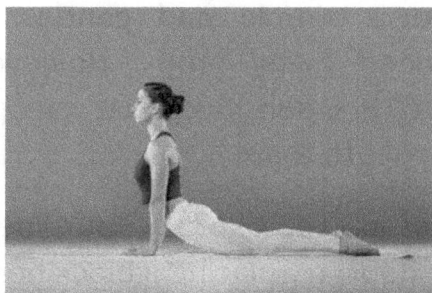

Instructions

Begin by lying face down on the floor on your mat. Place your hands palms down near your shoulders.

Use your arm strength to lift up your chest up, while flexing your legs.

Inhale to open your chest. Make sure your shoulders are moving down your back, not inching their way up to your ears.

Take about three breaths, then release the posture.

Add this posture into your vinyasa or do it three times in a row for an excellent stretch to your back.

Modifications

If you are too stiff and sore to lie face down on the ground, or if you are pregnant, you can do this posture standing up. Grasp the edge of a counter or a railing, and recreate the arch in your back.

Sphinx Pose

Sanskrit name: Salamba Bhujangasana

If you found that Cobra Pose was too intense for you, Sphinx Pose may be what you need instead. Sphinx pose is essentially a much less intense version of Cobra Pose, making it ideal for beginners or those struggling a lot with lower back pain.

This pose stretches out your back, stomach, chest, and shoulders. Since Sphinx Pose creates a stretch across the stomach, it can also be used to treat digestive discomforts from autoimmune disorders, overeating, bloating, or painkillers.

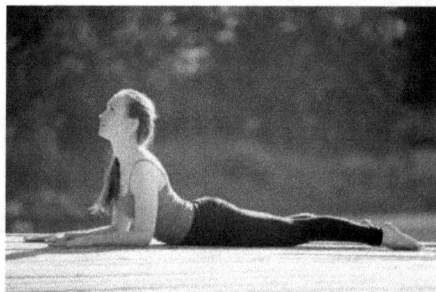

Instructions

Begin face down on your stomach on your mat. Place your hands flat on the ground beneath each shoulder, with your forearms resting in the ground.

Press the tops of your feet into the ground and lift up your chest, resting on your forearms.

Lower your shoulders down your back, rather than allowing them to move up towards your ears.

Breathe deep to open the chest and remain breathing in this pose for as long as needed.

Modifications

Avoid this pose if you are pregnant or recovering from abdominal or back surgery.

You can also perform this pose standing up straight behind a sturdy chair or railing. Grasp the back of the chair, arch your back, and move your chest forward in the same way you would if performing this pose on the floor.

Melting Heart Posture

Sanskrit name: Anahatasana

A lot of attention is paid to the lower back, and for good reason, because we tend to store tension and pain there. But since most of us sit behind a computer or the wheel of a car much more than we should, our upper and middle backs fall out of alignment and create pain for us. Melting

Heart Posture, or Puppy Dog Pose, might just be the ultimate tonic for pain caused by a sedentary lifestyle.

Bad posture and a sedentary lifestyle make arthritis pain much worse, and that's why so many doctors recommend yoga. This pose will bring flexibility to a stiff back while also opening the shoulders.

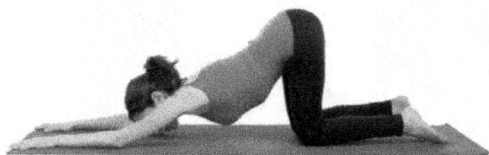

Instructions

Begin in tabletop pose, then walk your hands forward enough that your hips are still elevated while your chest is stretched towards the ground and your arms are forward.

While settling into the pose, feel free to move or sway the shoulders, upper body, and hips a little from side to side, for a bit of extra stretching and to find comfort and settle in.

Breathe while you hold this pose for up to six minutes.

Props

If this pose causes too much strain or hurts your neck, place a bolster under your chest so you can rest the body.

This pose may not best the best choice if you have arthritis in your knees. If this is the case, use a blanket or yoga gel pads under the knees to take the pressure off.

Modifications

If your shoulders are too tight, move your hands further apart.

For those with neck pain, this pose might put strain on the neck. If you want to relax your neck, put a bolster under your head or upper body. You can also fold one arm and rest your head on your forearm. If you choose this modification, just be sure to switch sides before ending the pose.

Rabbit Pose

Sanskrit name: Sasangasana

Rabbit Pose is another brilliant way to counteract the effects of sitting behind a desk all day. This calming posture creates a stretch from your lower back through your shoulders and neck, while dissipating tension and creating space in your intervertebral discs. However, if you are dealing with a lot of neck pain or have recently had surgery, you might want to skip this posture.

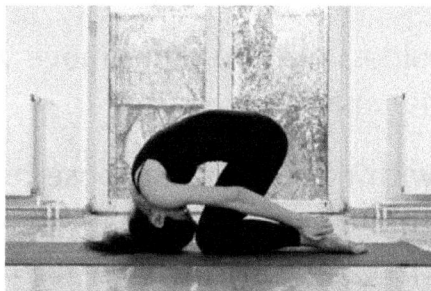

Instructions

Begin by sitting on your heels. Grab your feet with your fingertips pointing inwards and your thumbs on the outside of your feet.

While still grasping your feet, begin to roll forward until your hips are high, your back is rounded, and the crown of your head is touching the floor. You should still be holding on to your feet.

Make sure your shoulders are not inching up towards your ears, and breathe for as long as needed.

To exit the pose, slowly shift your weight back onto your feet, and bring your back up again, one vertebrae at a time. Do not move your neck until you are sitting completely erect.

Props

If you cannot reach your feet, loop a strap or a towel around your heels and hold on to that instead.

Since you will be resting on your knees, feel free to put a towel or a blanket under your knees.

Modifications

If you'd like to intensify the shoulder stretch, add a hand clasp behind your back. This modification will, however, put greater stress on the neck.

Holding lower on your feet can help relieve some of the pressure on your head.

Half Lord of the Fishes Pose

Sanskrit name: Ardha Matsyendrasana

Half Lord of the Fishes Pose is a gentle twist that brings relief to your lower back. It's similar to Bharadvaja's Twist, but much less intense, so if you found that twist to be too much, this pose can be a good alternative to, or even a preparation for, Bharadvaja's Twist.

This pose delivers all of the digestive benefits of a twist. It also wrings the tension out of the spine while stretching the neck, shoulders, and hips. For those who have severe back pain or have recently had back surgery, it might be best to skip this pose.

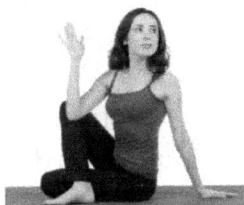

Instructions

Sit on your mat with your legs out straight in front of you, then bend your knees so your feet are flat on the ground, knees up.

Collapse your left leg onto the ground so your knee is still bent and your thigh is flush with the floor. Move your left foot close to your right buttock.

Place your right foot on the outside of your left leg, moving your left leg in closer to the body if needed.

Press your right arm behind your body, straight against your side, forcing you to sit upright.

Twist your entire upper body to the right, keeping your right arm straight. Look over your right shoulder.

Place your left elbow on the outside of your right leg. Your palm should be open and your hand facing upwards.

Breathe deeply to stretch your chest. Make sure your shoulders are moving down your back not creeping up your neck.

Props

You can also try this pose seated in a chair if your hips are tight. Grasp the back of the chair with your right hand and twist to the right. Repeat on the other side. Breathe deeply, allowing the breath to move in and out naturally with the twist.

Modifications

If you're dealing with a sore or weak back, practice this pose against the wall.

If your shoulders are very tight, this pose can be practiced with just the twist, leaving out the arm posture.

Tree Pose

Sanskrit name: Vrksasana

One of the most important things for preventing back pain is developing strong lower back and abdominal muscles. If your arthritis is severe or you're a beginner to yoga, you might not be ready for an intense ab workout.

Balancing poses are a great alternative because they help to gently strengthen your core. Tree Pose in particular is especially helpful for those suffering from arthritis because it also opens the chest and the hips.

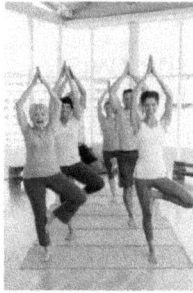

Instructions

Begin standing upright in Mountain Pose.

Shift your weight to your right foot.

Bend your left knee and lift it upwards as much as you can. You might not be able to get your foot completely off of the ground.

Turn your knee outwards so your legs create a figure four. Place your foot flat against your right ankle, calf, or inner thigh. Do not rest your foot against your knee. Activate your core to maintain your balance.

Sweep your hands overhead and place your palms together. Leave them here, or bring them down into Prayer Hands against your chest or Reverse Prayer Hands against your back.

Hold the pose for a few breaths, and then switch sides.

Props

If you are unable to balance, try this pose next to a chair. Grasp the back of the chair with your right hand while you balance on your right foot, then switch sides.

Modifications

If you're working on the balancing portion, but don't feel completely comfortable, practice this pose near a wall. If you start to fall you can reach out to the wall for support.

If balancing is not an option for you, try this pose reclining on the ground. Lie down on your back and create a figure four with your legs by placing the left foot flat against your inner thigh. Let the knee fall outwards, if you can. If this is too intense of a hip and thigh stretch, place

the foot against your right ankle. Repeat
on the other side.

Chapter 11: Yoga Exercises For Stress

There are many different poses that will help you with stress levels and you will learn which ones help you the most. Although we have a chapter on poses, I thought that singling out a pose that works particularly well for stress would be a good idea. This pose is one such pose. As the above quotation states, yoga is all about energy, so don't just do one pose as that limits you. Try to incorporate different poses into your routine because this helps you to develop bodily curve and perfect harmony within yourself.

The pose that I want to introduce for stress is the Adhomukha Savasana. People know this as the "Downward facing dog" and there's something to be said for using this pose to gain humility and humility helps stress levels. Some people actually see humility as a weakness though I and many other philosophers see it as a great human strength. If you know how to be humble, you also know how to appreciate things and see the world from a different perspective — one that has few expectations but that gains much just through that observation. Humility is one of the most powerful spiritual feelings that a human can experience so don't underestimate it.

Adhomukha Savasana

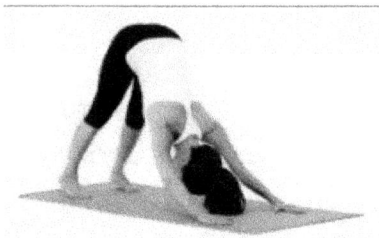

For this pose you need to be suitable attired. Don't wear anything that is constrictive. If you are wearing shorts make sure that they are ones that have an elasticated waistband. The idea of the pose is not to make you uncomfortable or restricted. Kneel on the mat and lean forward so that your palms are on the mat at shoulder width. You will need to have your palms downward to support you. Move up onto your feet and position your hip area just above where your feet are placed on the mat.

Inhale and pull your tummy upward so that your body forms an upside down V. Exhale and move your tailbone so that it is pointing to the sky. While you are in this position, inhale and exhale about four or five times, keeping your legs straight and your arms straight and making sure that your tailbone is as high as possible. Feeling the body stretch and this exercise is a very good one for making you feel energized. Exhale and go back to your kneeling position and relax, hands stretched out in front of you. Inhale and keep this position for three breaths. Exhale and move back to your original position and relax.

There's something that you should note about yoga by now, even though you are new to it. The inhale and exhale are used to spur movements or to reinforce a position once you are in it. Think of breath as being energy. Instead of thinking "I can't do this" think in terms of the breath allowing you that extra bit of energy that enables you to do it.

You may struggle with this exercise at first but it really is a good exercise to help you to learn to be more flexible and to allow the flow within your body to be constant. What flow is that? Well, your body has a series of points that are called chakras. These are located around the different parts of the body and if these are blocked, then energy fails to be able to flow. If you imagine them as junction points – for the body to perform at optimal levels, each junction point should be open so that the energy can go through it to the next junction point. This exercise is a good one for opening up the flow along the spine, in the chest area and up through the neck. It's particularly good for concentration because of its inverted nature.

When you are doing this exercise, you find that you don't think of other things because you are too immersed in getting the exercise right. If you can practice and have a mirror so that you can see your own body straightness down the two sides of the inverted V, this will help you to get your tailbone into the right position so that your yoga session is more complete and you actually achieve something from the downward dog pose.

Chapter 12: Getting Deeper Into The Practice

Now that you've understood the Seven Chakras and how they impact your weight, you can begin to achieve a state of balance.

Firstly, make a commitment to spend the first couple of hours in the morning pursuing your weight loss routine. For this, you need to regulate the rest of your lifestyle by getting to bed earlier in order to get six to eight hours of sleep each night. Begin the day with a glass of warm water with the juice of one lemon and a teaspoon of honey.

Find yourself a spot outdoors if possible or practice Yoga in a well ventilated space indoors.

It's important at this time to keep your mind free of everything barring what you are doing. Focus on the practice and not on your weight or what you need to accomplish during the day.

Warm up exercises:

Begin by rotating your head from side to side – slowly and deliberately, touching your right ear to your right shoulder, bringing your head down to your chest, touching your left ear to your left shoulder, and bending your head back as far as it will go.

Now place your left hand on your right shoulder, extend your arm and rotate it over your shoulder backwards and forwards, at least five times each. Switch to placing your right hand on your left shoulder, stretching and rotating your left arm over your shoulder from front to back and then from back to front, at least five times each.

Place your hands on your shoulders – right hand on right shoulder and left hand on left shoulder, and rotate your shoulders from front to back and back to front, with your elbows extended.

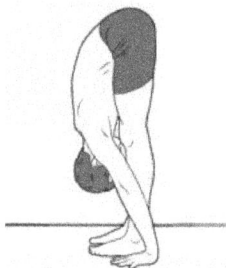

Now place your hands on your hips and begin to rotate your lower body moving from right to left and then from left to right. Make sure you thrust out your pelvis as you rotate your hips forward, and push your bottom out when you rotate your hips towards the back. Repeat this at least ten times in each direction (left to right and right to left), and move slowly and deliberately.

Standing with your feet slightly apart, stretch your arms with palms facing forward and fingers pointing upwards. Bring your arms forward with the palms coming together but not touching. Inhale deeply as you widen your arms, and exhale as you bring them together in front of your chest. This exercise strengthens your lungs and chest muscles.

Breathe in deeply through your nose while holding your arms up against your chest, hands folded into fists. Exhale in a gust through your mouth with a **"ho"** as you throw your hands out straight in front of you, with the fingers of both your hands bent tight like claws. Repeat this five times.

Bend over and, with your knees absolutely straight and feet together, place your hands, palms down on the floor on either side of your feet. If you can't do this, then touch your toes. Remain in this position for ten slow counts.

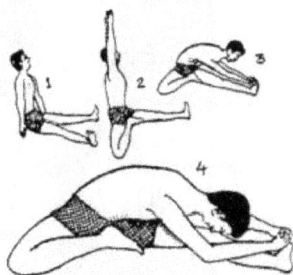

Sit down and extend your legs in front of you. Fold your left leg up so that your left foot is pressed against your right thigh, with the heel of your left foot touching the highest point of your right thigh. Clutch the toes of your right foot with both hands and pull them back towards you as you lower your forehead to touch your right leg. Release your legs from this position and then fold your right leg up so that your right foot is pressed against your left thigh with the heel of your right foot touching the highest point of your left thigh. Then clutch the toes of your left foot with both hands, and pull them back towards you as you lower your forehead to touch your left leg. Feel the stretch in your hamstrings and spine.

You will find this a little difficult to accomplish when you first get started, but with practice you will be able to go into this posture with ease.

Strong spine, supple body with Marjariasana - Cat Cow Pose

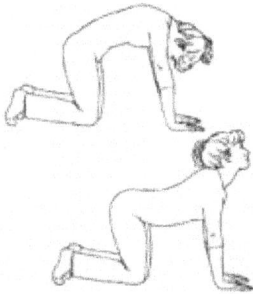

Start by kneeling on your hands and knees, and gaze at a spot on the floor about three feet in front of you. Make sure your knees are in line with your hips and wrists, and that your elbows and shoulders are perpendicular to the floor.

Inhale and slowly round your spine toward the ceiling. Drop your head toward the floor. This is the Cat Pose.

Exhale and slowly bring your spine back to starting position returning your gaze to the original spot.

Now inhale and lift both your chest and tailbone to the ceiling while curving your back down towards the floor. Raise your head up but do not force it back. This is the Cow Pose.

Exhale and slowly bring your spine back to starting position.

Repeat this for ten slow counts. This practice improves flexibility and abdominal strength.

The benefits of Marjariasana

It works on your spine to keep it strong and supple. (Imagine if your spine was in poor shape. It would slow you down and keep you from shedding weight.)

Stimulates internal organs so that your digestion and circulation is super-efficient

It relieves stress so that you are calm in mind and body and don't keep reaching for fattening comfort foods

It improves posture and balance – so important for your image

As a bonus, it also tones your reproductive organs

Chapter 13: Lying Down And The Shoulderstand Cycle

The Corpse Pose

This is a kind of pose that many yogi use at the beginning of each session. Its main purpose is to prepare you both physically and mentally for the big work ahead. The corpse pose is also done after each position as a way of releasing energy to flow freely and drive out waste from the body. You may hold to this pose for five minutes before and after you begin the session, and for a few minutes in between each pose.

How to do it:

Lie on your back with relax toes, legs apart, and fingers curled gently. The arms must be 45 degrees to the body. Close your eyes and lie still.

The Single Leg Lift

Start with your legs as straight as possible and your feet flexed. Lift each leg for three times. As you lift your leg, synchronize the movement with your breath.

How to do it:

Lie flat on your back with your feet together and both hands on the side. Inhale as you lift your left leg, and then exhale as you lower your leg. Repeat the same procedure for the other leg.

The Double Leg Lift

This specific position requires a stronger lumbar and abdominal muscles as compared to the single leg lift. You may control the movement by doing proper breathing.

How to do it:

Lie flat on your back and inhale as you slowly bring your legs up. Then, exhale as you lower your legs. Remember to keep your legs and knees straight, arms on the side, and do not let your back arch. You may begin with five lifts and build up to 10 if you can.

The Fish

This particular position comes from the corpse pose. It relieves tension in the shoulders, neck and throat. It also tones the abdominals and relieves stress and tension.

How to do it:

Lie flat on your back and keep your legs straight. Tuck your arms under your body and tilt your head until the crown reaches the floor. Inhale as you arch your chest upward. Hold to the position for 30 seconds.

The Shoulderstand Cycle is one yoga pose that helps toughen the muscles, improves spine flexibility, and aids in balancing the thyroid glands.

The Shoulderstand

This pose stretches your upper back muscles.

Word of caution: For beginners, do not force yourself into a position you feel you cannot perform. Do this with the help of an instructor.

How to do it:

Lie on your back with arms on the side, palms facing down and feet together. Breathe in as you raise your legs to a 90-degree angle.

Next, place your hands on your buttocks and exhale as you raise your body by walking your hands up your back until you rest on your shoulders.

As you hold to the position for 30 seconds, remember to breathe normally.

To come down, exhale as you drop your feet half way. Place your hands flat on the floor below your back, and then gradually unfold your body.

The Plow

This is the position following the shoulderstand. It increases your overall flexibility and releases tension in the shoulders and upper back. In this pose, you are required that your feet touch the floor behind your head to create a bending of the spine. If while practicing you feel your legs tense up, do not continue.

You may do the following instead:

In a lying position, inhale as you support your back, and exhale as you lower your legs.

Keep the knees straight as you lift them up above your head. If your toes cannot reach the floor, you may choose to rest your knees on your forehead instead.

The Bridge

This is a position that comes after the Plow. This provides a balancing stretch of the lumbar and thoracic regions.

How to do it:

From the corpse position, bend your knees with your two feet flat on the ground. Place your hands on your back with the fingers pointing down the spine. Your feet must remain flat whilst your head and shoulders rest on the floor.

Chapter 14: The Postmodern Predicament

WHERE HAVE ALL THE FLOWER CHILDREN GONE?

When we or our parents were young, forty-five years ago, there were flower children in the streets and they were all going to have an everlasting love-in. Well, that failed and it's kind of embarrassing to recall, to tell you the truth. Certainly the kids today think it was kind of naive or worse. They snicker. There were gurus on every corner and people practiced Eastern ways and meditated and took LSD and chanted, "Hell no, we won't go!"

Today's child, a member of whatever the latest generation calls itself, works for a corporation making products and schemes and proprietary software to seduce a witless population, sodas and cigarettes, television fantasies and insurance frauds. Everything we touch today is more or less corrupt. If we weren't working for MegaFraud Insurance we might be working for a corporation that sells deodorants by making people afraid they smell bad or for a tobacco company that still sees no link between its product and cancer or for a garment manufacturer that exploits child labor overseas. It's not easy to see where virtue ends and the corruption begins, and since corruption is everywhere maybe it's not corruption at all but the natural scheme of things.

All is relative and all ways of knowing are just social constructions shaped by the ever winding, ever clever river of the zeitgeist.

The average person of today doesn't believe in gurus and can't spare the time to meditate.

But our average person as usual is wrong. And we know it. The tide of pollution, the escalation of dependencies of all kinds, the obesity, the growing number of hungry and homeless persons even in our own very rich society (to say nothing of Africa and India), the rise of a mindless terrorism, the continued addiction by many to a false fundamentalism, all attest mightily to the fact that we are lost and desperately need to be found.

We tried yoga once, actually, when we were younger. We needed to relax, we were so uptight all the time. But we lost confidence in the practice because how much faith can you have in something that claims to cure all disease? And take a look at India would you? If yoga's so good how come life in India is so bad? The question fairly begging for an answer here is why should we have the slightest interest in yoga?

ANCIENT INDIA

There is no way in a few words (or even in many words) that I or anyone else can satisfactory answer that question. It is only through the practice of yoga that the answer can be found. But I think I can hint at the answer here in this chapter. At least

I hope that I can offer some compelling rationale for turning to yoga. At the very least I can point.

While many of our postmodern problems are unique to our time and place, our basic predicament has not changed in ten thousand years. In fact, our situation is the same today as it was when we still lived in tribes on the savannas and in the primordial forest. Instinctively we know there can be no escape from the sadness of life until we find ourselves and are reunited with the Ineffable.

In ancient India before recorded history there grew up a civilization along the banks of the inland rivers of the Indus Valley. The land was especially fertile and people had just arrived at agriculture. For numerous centuries, some say perhaps five thousand years, there existed a civilization comprised of millions of people. This was one of the first great societies of the world. And during those many years (far more than during all of the experience of recorded history) people had time to contemplate their existence and had ample opportunity to share their conclusions with others. During this period there were no ancient texts to advise the people on how to live. There was no medical science or social science or mathematics or any of the vast learning we have today that helps us to shape our lives and guide us. There was only human instinct and the social ways of the tribe. Instead of the church there was the shaman. Instead of the teacher there was the mother and father, grandparents, and perhaps the aunt and uncle or the guru. Knowledge grew slowly, by word of mouth, handed down from parent to child. Basic ideas that we take for granted were actually composed in those days, ideas such as the need for cleanliness, for prayer, what was good to eat, what was not, how to behave, what to do and what not to do. Innumerable practices and ideas were tried and discarded, some to be taken up again and discarded again. Some practices (like fertilizing the fields, for example) were shown after a long trial to be essential and became the conventional wisdom and the standard practice. Science itself was still just sympathetic magic.

Society was mixed and remixed; the gene pool stirred mightily for hundreds of generations. All manner of social and sexual practices were tried. Trade developed. People learned how to live together. They learned how to follow the seasons and avoid the worst of the parasites. Yoga was born.

Many yogas were born, actually. They were all tried and tested. People compared experience and knowledge. Centuries passed. Certain practices, **asanas** (postures), **pranayamas** (breathing exercises), diets, etc., were shown to be efficacious. These practices for harmonious living were polished and re-polished, improved upon and built upon until a vast knowledge was accumulated. This knowledge was honed and committed to memory and finally codified and systematized and at last written down.

THE UNCHANGING NATURE OF THE HUMAN CONDITION

Since then, during the 2,000 or so years that have passed since Patanjali wrote his **Yoga Sutras**, yoga has spread throughout the world. Great religions have taken up many of its ideas. Secular schools based on its practices have sprung up in our great cities.

All of this has taken thousands of years. The yogas that grew out of this vast social and existential, this vast political and physical experience, were directed toward solving essentially the same problems that people face today. Nothing important has changed. We still don't know where we came from or why. We don't know the meaning of life (or whether life has a meaning or whether such a word as "meaning" might apply). We live a little longer but still die after around three score and ten. We still suffer from disease and psychological pain. We still have to get up in the morning and go to sleep at night. We still have sex and see our children grow up. We're still subject to anger and hate, love and the finality of death. Nothing important has changed. Our psychological condition is the same.

So the question is asked: Does the yoga that millions of people have developed over countless billions of hours have any relevance for us today? It would be a foolish person who misses the overwhelmingly clear answer. That answer is yes.

Chapter 15: Plank Pose

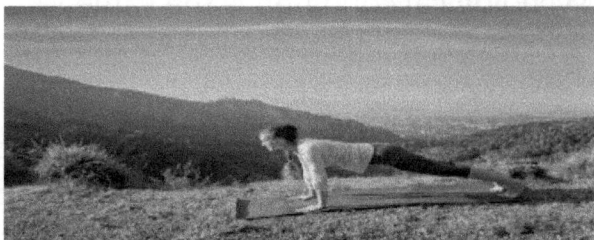

Plank Pose is another key staple in any regular yoga practitioner's repertoire. Also known as 'Phalakasana,' it forms a solid basis for many other stretches. It is a good exercise for strengthening core abdominal muscles and building a stronger back. This in turn will improve your posture. Begin in 'Downward-Facing Dog' as described in the previous chapter. Inhale, and move your body forward. You need to align your arms so that they are perpendicular with the floor, with your wrists and shoulders lined up, and your torso running parallel to the ground. Press your palms into the floor, pushing through the bases of your fingers. Inhale and spread your shoulders, ensuring that they are not hunched, tensed or rounded. Your gaze should be directed straight down towards the floor. Keep your breathing soft and even. Lengthen your spine. Hold this pose for 40-60 seconds.

Boat Pose

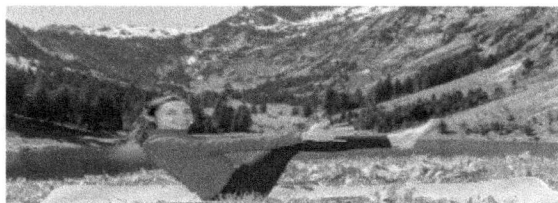

Boat Pose ('Paripurna Navasana') is named after the position your body adopts once you have moved into the pose. Done correctly, the practitioner slightly resembles a sailboat. This asana is good for building core strength and tight abdominal muscles. It also promotes balance and general flexibility.

Lie down on the floor, flat on your back. Place your legs and ankles together so that they are lightly touching. Inhale deeply. As you exhale, smoothly lift your feet and torso from the floor. Keeping your fingers together and wrists relaxed, extend your arms towards your feet. Aim to keep your toes, fingers and eyes in alignment. If you are doing this pose correctly, you should feel the muscles in your abdomen tense. Your torso and legs should be at an approximate angle of 45 degrees. This is a great sign that this asana is strengthening your core, which in turn will promote good posture.

Hold this pose for 15-30 seconds. To exit the pose, exhale and lower your legs back to the floor. As you become more accomplished at Boat Pose, you can try holding it for longer periods of time during your yoga sessions.

Happy Baby Pose

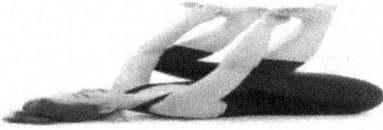

The Happy Baby Pose is named after a position we've all seen many young babies adopt! Otherwise known as 'Ananda Balasana,' this pose is good for improving hip flexibility, for stretching the muscles in your back, and even alleviating mild lower back pain.

Lie down on the floor, flat on your back. Take a few deep breaths. As you exhale, bring your knees up to your abdomen. On your next inhalation, take hold of the outer edges of each foot with the corresponding hand - right hand to right foot, left hand to left foot. Spread your knees slightly so that they are a little wider apart in comparison to your shoulders. Stay in this pose for 30-60 seconds. To exit the pose, exhale and gently lower your feet back to the floor.

If you find it difficult to maintain a firm hold on your feet, you can loop a yoga strap around them instead and hold onto that instead. If you find that your neck feels especially tense in this pose, fold a blanket into a square several inches thick and rest your head on it whilst carrying out this asana.

Standing Forward Bend

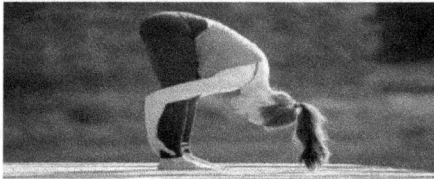

Standing Forward Bend ('Uttanasana') really stretches out tense muscles in your legs, especially your hamstrings. It also has a calming effect on the body as a whole.

Begin by standing on the floor with your feet together. Bending from your hips rather than your lower back, bend your knees and fold your body over your legs. Position your hands, palms down, on the tops of your feet or alongside them on the ground. Look forward whilst in this pose. Taking a deep breath in, push out your chest and lengthen your back. Take another breath, and as you exhale straighten your legs as much as possible without causing yourself undue pain or discomfort.

Take another breath and this time when you exhale, extend your body down over your legs towards the floor. Do not round your shoulders - draw them back towards your back instead. Do not allow your head to hang limply - keep your neck muscles engaged and the crown of your head drawn towards the ground. If you find it difficult to reach your feet or the ground with your hands, you can use props to enhance you experience of this pose. You could use a yoga strap looped around your feet and hold onto that, or else you could rest your hands on foam yoga blocks placed close by on the floor.

Chapter 16: Yoga And Meditation

Meditation is a yogic exercise that gives you deep rest, which is far from what you get when you sleep daily. Meditation is when and where the mind is free from all forms of agitation. It is calm and peaceful and when in peace, meditation happens. Resting in meditation is more relaxing than the most comfortable sleep you ever could have.

The benefits of meditation are widely known and extremely crucial. Meditation is a necessary form of exercise for maintenance of mental health. A relaxed mind with proper focus and clear thoughts and enhanced communication are some of the results of meditation. Other benefits of meditation include springing skills and talents with powerful cognizant strength, the ability to associate with a greater and deeper form of energy, and rejuvenation.

Here are a few yoga postures, which you can practice during meditation to make the meditation process much easier and more effective.

These yogic meditation postures are very effective tools for peaceful and successful meditation. They assist the human body and mind in relaxing the nervous system as well as in acquiring and accomplishing physical, mental, emotional, and spiritual balance.

Padmasana

This posture is also known as Lotus Pose among yoga experts. Start by being in the sitting position and gradually place your right foot onto your left thigh. After this, take hold of your left foot and carefully place it onto the right thigh. Keep breathing in deeply and exhaling out with force. Keep the body as straight as possible with both knees in contact with the floor. Place the palms of your hands or just the wrists on your knees, or rest the hands between the heels or make the right hand rest on the left hand.

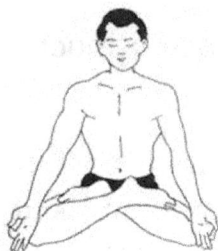

Siddhasana

This posture is also known as Adepts Pose. Start from the sitting position and bend your left leg while placing the heel at the perineum. Then, bend the right leg and position the heel against the pubic bone, or just above the genital region. This pose is held by keeping the body as erect as possible with the hands placed in a similar manner like that of Padmasana.

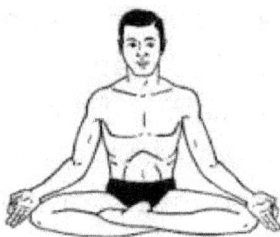

Swastikasana

This yoga posture is not well known as the Ankle lock Pose rather it is by its generic name, Swastikasana. The word 'Swastika' in Sanskrit translates to prosperous thereby implying that it showers prosperity, success, and good health to the one who practices it. It is done by extending the legs right in front. Then, you bend the right leg at the knee and the right heel is positioned against the groin of the left thigh. This is done so as to ensure that the sole will be able to touch the thigh. Similarly, bend the left leg and place it against the right groin. Then enclose the toes of your left foot between the right calf and thigh muscles. After this sort of positioning, both feet are seen to lie in between the calves and thigh muscles. Place the hands in a manner similar to that of Padmasana.

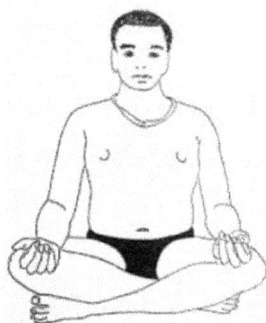

Sukhasana

This posture is one of the simplest in yogic meditation and is hence referred to as, Easy Pose. This asana is achieved by simply crossing the legs and keeping the head and trunk straight at an angle of 90 degrees. The hands are placed in a manner similar to that of Padmasana.

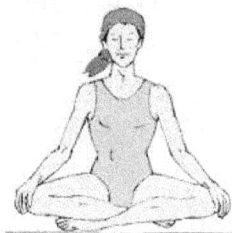

For inculcating the process of meditation, you have to go through few checkpoints before you jump into the main event unprepared. Here are a few tips for beginners in the field of yogic meditation.

#Take deep breathes

Yoga is all about a simple process of uniting yourself – your soul and body together by using your breath, body, and the mind.

#Simple wearing, high thinking

Comfortable clothing or clothing you feel relaxed in is ideal for a yoga class or even while practicing yoga at home, as it does not block your progress. Avoid excess jewelry and belts since this can make you uncomfortable or even obstruct your yoga practice.

#Lighter stomach aids to your yoga practice

Yoga on an empty stomach or at least 2-3 hours after your last meal is more effective and accurate. Drink lots of water and eat light food.

#Set the tone right before you start

Casual warm up exercises will loosen up the body early to prepare you for the strenuous yoga postures to come.

#Smile

See the difference in yourself when you keep a gentle smile, which relaxes the body and mind and helps you benefit from the yoga postures.

There are certain rules you need to follow before you meditate, and after you meditate to make the most of the time you spent meditating.

Before Meditation

-It is advisable to cleanse yourself by taking a shower and wearing a fresh pair of clothes to begin your session of meditation.

-Settling down to rest for meditation is extremely important for the mind. If you have extra five minutes, you would want to stretch your muscles through a quick warm-up followed by a few yoga asanas or a few sets of Suryanamaskar Kriya.

-Empty stomach meditation is always preferred. Eating a meal might block the efficiency of your meditation as your body and mind aren't relaxed but are in a continuous state of work.

After Meditation

-A few minutes of silence after a session is recommended for digestion of thoughts and processes. It is not recommended to rush to your computer and television immediately after meditation. Get back to your work gradually, building a momentum. Sudden jerk of activity could be tasking.

-You will feel hungry after your meditation. Have something fresh once you finish your meditation to quench your hunger. Repeat the meal pattern for the evening meditation.

Chapter 17: Yoga Poses To Boost Your Immunity

While there are many yoga poses that can help boost your immunity, in this section, we will be discussing four key poses for achieving this end.

The Cobra Pose

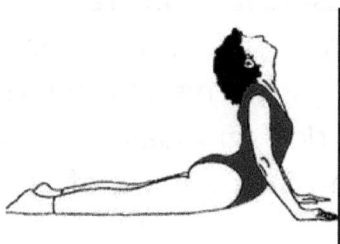

This pose is ideal for stimulating the thymus, the organ located at the back of your chest bone that regulates the growth of the cells that control the outbreak of flu and cold.

How to go about the pose:

Lie on your stomach with your feet and legs straightened behind you☐

Place your two palms on the floor with your fingers pointing in front of you ☐

Tuck your elbows close to your body ☐

Close your eyes and relax with your head resting on the floor☐

Using your back muscles, slowly raise your head, your neck, and then your shoulders from the floor☐

Keep your pubic bone resting on the floor while lifting your torso with your arm muscles ☐

Lengthen and strengthen your spine into a backward curve and keep your gaze upwards.☐

Hold this pose for as long as you can, then release slowly by bending the elbows, lowering the chest, navel, shoulders, and finally your forehead towards the floor ☐

Inhale while raising your torso☐

Exhale while lowering your torso☐

You can practice this pose for about ten rounds. ☐

The Downward Facing Dog Pose

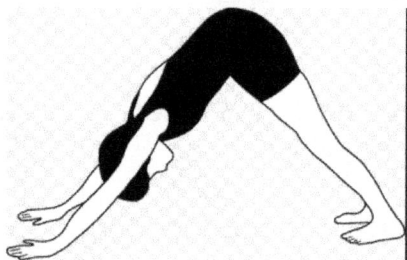

This yoga pose is ideal for when you feel overwhelmed and when things seem to be moving rapidly out of control. Placing a block under your forehead will increase your feeling of restoration and calmness.

This pose provides you grounded energy and enhanced circulation. The downward dog pose is also ideal for draining congested sinuses and strengthening your immune system.

How to go about this pose:

Go down on all fours with your knees set directly below your hips and kept slightly forward from your shoulders. Keep your palms extended with your index finger slightly turned out or parallel and your toes turned under ☐

As you exhale, lift your knees off the floor. At first, keep the knees slightly bent with your heels lifted off the floor. Keep your tailbone lengthened away from the back of your pelvic region and keep it lightly pressed towards the pubis ☐

Lift the sitting bones a bit towards the ceiling then draw the inner legs up into the groins from the inner ankle ☐

As you exhale, push back your top thighs and push your heels down towards the floor. Keep your knees straightened while ensuring they are not locked together. Keep your outer thighs firm and slightly roll your upper thighs inwards and then narrow the front side of your pelvic region☐

Keep your outer arms firm and the bases of your index fingers actively pressed into the floor; from these points, lift with your inner arms from your wrists towards the top of your shoulders. Keep the shoulder blades firmed against your back as you widen and draw them in the direction of your tailbone. Keep the head in between the upper arms. ☐

You can maintain this pose from 1-3 minutes while practicing deep/abdominal breathing and end by bending your knees towards the floor, exhale and rest in the "child pose."☐

Legs on the Wall

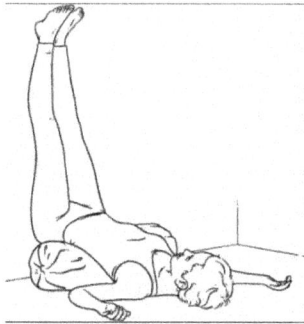

This yoga pose is the go-to pose for grounding the nervous system. This pose will not only boost your immunity, it will also drastically reduce your stress levels. As you engage in this yoga pose, your body pumps highly oxygenated blood to your two legs, which brings a deep feeling of calmness and helps revive your tired muscles.

How to go about this pose:

Experiment with the distance from the wall to find a distance most suitable for you height □

You can begin with your support placed about 5-6 inches from the wall. Sit on the right end of your support with your right side placed against the wall. With one smooth movement, lift your legs onto the wall with your head and shoulders lightly placed on the floor ☐

Your sitting bone should be between the wall and the support. Make sure the top of your torso arches gently from your pubis to the top of your shoulders ☐

Lift the base of your skull away from the back of your neck to soften your throat. Ensure your chin does not push against your sternum. However, you can lift your sternum towards your chin. Open the shoulder blades away from the spine and then release the arms and hands out to the sides, and the palms lifted up. ☐

Ensure to keep the legs firm enough to ensure you keep them vertically in place. Then release the head of your thighbones using the weight of the belly deeply into the torso close to the back of the pelvic region. ☐

You can hold this pose from 5-15 minutes. Bend your knees and keep your feet pressed against the wall as you lift your pelvis off the support. You can then slide the support to one side before lowering your pelvis to the floor. Turn to the side and hold for a few breaths before coming up to a sitting position as you exhale. □

Supported Fish Pose

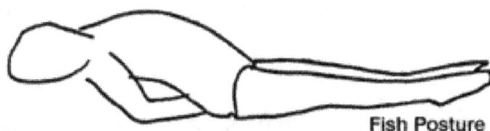

Fish Posture

The supported Fish Pose is a restorative and invigorating pose that opens up the lungs and heart and breaks up the congestion in your sinuses and lungs. The fish pose helps you access deep/abdominal breath and helps balance your nervous system when it is agitated.

How to go about this pose:

Place your block at the bottom tips of your shoulder blades. Make sure your neck has a gentle natural curve with adequate support from the second block ☐

Lie with your feet on the floor and your knees bent. Lift your pelvis off the floor as you inhale. Slide your palms below your buttocks, keep your buttocks resting at the back of your hands, and leave them there while you perform this pose. Make sure that the elbows and forearms remain properly tucked upwards close to the torso☐

Firmly press your elbows and forearms against the floor. Then keep your scapulae pressed into your back, and as you exhale, lift the head and the upper torso away from the floor ☐

You can keep your legs straightened or your knees bent. If you choose to keep your legs straightened, make sure your thigh is active and pressed out through your heels ☐

Hold for 15-30 seconds' time during which you should breathe deeply and smoothly. With each exhalation, keep your torso and head lowered towards the floor then lift your thighs upwards into your belly as you squeeze. ☐

Yoga Poses for Building Stamina

Yoga is a great relaxation tool, which can help you to distress, build your strength and relax irrespective of your work environment. In fact, by practicing yoga, it becomes easier to be fully focused on your work thus enhancing productivity.

Here are some poses that you can practice building your stamina.

Boat Pose

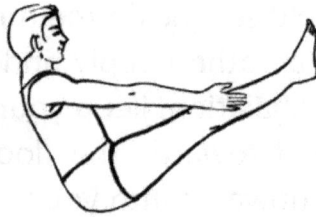

This is a basic yoga asana known to help you achieve a much stronger core.

How to go about this pose:

Sit on the floor with bent knees. Place your hands around your hip area ☐

Gently inhale and exhale☐

Straighten your spine☐

Lean back and lift your feet from the floor☐

Keep your shins parallel to the floor☐

Now bring your arms forward☐

Maintain a straightened spine and keep the lower part of your belly flat and firm☐

Focus your gaze on your toes and try to relax. Maintain this position for 5 seconds or more and hold the pose for one minute☐

Release and repeat the entire process ☐

The Goddess Pose

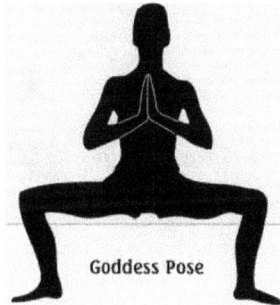

Goddess Pose

The Goddess Yoga pose is ideal for building your physical strength and stamina. It also reduces menstrual pains.

How to go about this pose:

Stand erect and keep your feet apart☐

Make sure your feet are facing sideways☐

Keep your two legs bent☐

Roll back downwards ☐

Lie down on your back while you keep your legs bent☐

This is a popular pose used by most pregnant women to help them stay strong on their feet. However, it is ideal for everyone irrespective of sex and age.

The Bridge Pose

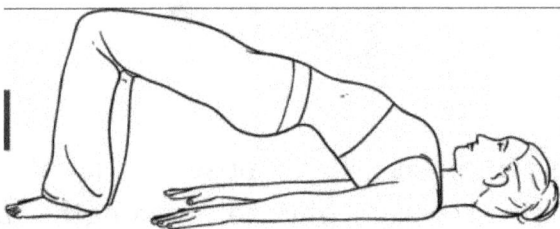

The bridge pose is ideal for toning your pelvic muscles and for keeping you strong and fit.

How to go about this pose:

Lie down on your yoga mat ☐

Keep your knees bent □

Lift the buttocks very gently until your two thighs are parallel to the floor and forms a bridge □

Stay in this position from 30-60 minutes and practice deep breathing □

Repeat the entire process □

Yoga Poses for Stress Management

The yoga poses in this section will wash away all your stress:

Child's Pose

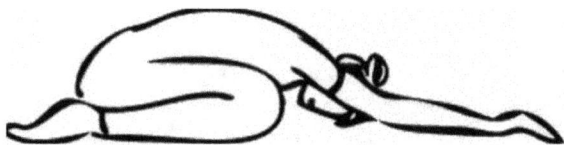

The child's pose keeps your senses, body, and mind relaxed. It is very effective at combating stress and improving work productivity. The child pose is a great stress buster you do not want to do without.

How to go about this pose:☐

Kneel on your yoga mat and slightly arch your back ☐

Bring both arms together and keep them stretched out before you☐

Rest your two palms on the floor☐

Hold for about 10 seconds, breath in deeply and repeat the process ☐

Corpse Pose

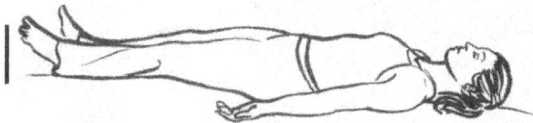

Because the corpse pose is a yoga pose that can guarantee you total relaxation anytime, many yogis use it to end their yoga exercise.

How to go about the corpse pose:

Lie on your back on your yoga mat without any cushions or supports—If need be, however, you can use a small pillow and then shut your eyes ☐

Keep your legs apart allowing your knees and feet to relax with your toes facing sideways ☐

Keep your arms on the sides, and spread them a little bit away from your body; face your palms upward ☐

Relax your whole body by focusing on various parts of your body one after the other.☐

Start with your right foot, bring awareness to it, and move to your right knee. Move to the left leg once done with the right leg. Continue until you get to the crown of your head. As you focus on each body part, it will relax☐

As you do this, breathe deeply and slowly, and let your deep gentle breaths help you relax more☐

Your body shall energize as you inhale and relax as you exhale. Be present with your breath and body and forget everything else ☐

To feel completely relaxed, hold the pose for 10-20 minutes before rolling to your right side. Lie quietly on your right side and maintain that position for 1-3 minutes, then support yourself with one hand and sit up. ☐

With your eyes still shut, take a couple of deep breaths and gradually become aware of your body and environment. To end the yoga session, mindfully open your eyes. ☐

Happy Baby Pose

The baby pose is a pose that helps you combat anxiety, depression, and stress.

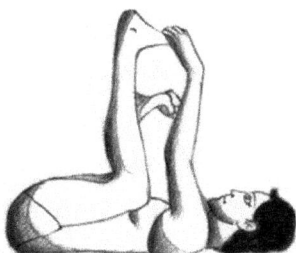

How to go about the baby pose:

Lie on your back and exhale as you bend the knees into the belly ☐

While inhaling, ensure to grip each foot with one hand. Keep your knees open a bit wider than your torso, and then pull them up in the direction of your armpits ☐

Keep each ankle directly positioned over your knee to keep your shins perpendicular to the floor while you flex through your heels. Very gently push your feet up into your hands and pull down your hands to create a resistance. ☐

Hold for 5-10 deep breaths before you release yourself from this position. ☐

150

Chapter 18: Yoga Poses For Stress & Anxiety Free Life

These yoga postures can help in achieving a happy and healthy mind and body. It also help you release tensions and negativity from the system.

1) Cat Stretch (Marjariasana)

Instructions to perform this pose:

Step-1: First step is to come onto your fours. Now Form a table such that your back forms the table top and your hands and feet form the legs of the table.

Step-2: Now keep your arms perpendicular to the floor, with the hands directly under the shoulders and flat on the ground; your knees should be hip-width apart.

Step-3: Look straight ahead.

Step-4: While inhaling raise your chin and tilt your head back, push your navel downwards and raise your tailbone.

Compress your buttocks. You will feel a slight tingle here.

Step-5: Maintain this pose and keep your breath even, deep and smooth.

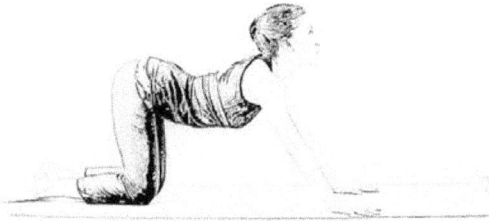

Fig. 2.1 Cat Pose

Step-6: Now while exhaling drop your chin to your chest and arch your back up as much as you can. Relax the buttocks.

Step-7: Maintain this pose for a few seconds and then come back to the initial table-like stage.

Step-8: Do five or six rounds of this pose for better results.

Beginner's Tip:

1. If you do the movement slowly and gracefully, its effect is more powerful and meditative.

Precautions:

1. If you have back or neck-related problems then consult your doctor before practicing this pose.

Other benefits:

1. This pose is practiced to help strengthen wrists and shoulders.

2. This pose improves digestion and massages productive organs.

2) Corpse Pose (Shavasana)

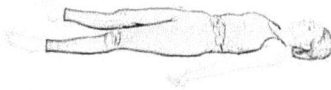

Fig. 2.2 Corpse Pose

Instructions to perform this pose:

Step-1: First of all lie flat on your back. Close your eyes. If required put small pillow below your neck.

Step-2: Now keep your legs comfortable apart and let your feet and knees relax completely, toes facing to the sides.

Step-3: Place your arms alongside, yet a little spread apart from your body. Leave your palms open, facing upward.

Step-4: Now take your attention to your body part by part and slowly relax your entire body.

Step-5: Start with bringing your awareness to the right foot, move on to the right knee (when you complete one leg, move your attention on to the other leg), and so on, and slowly move upwards to your head, relaxing every part of your body.

Step-6: Keep your breath smooth, deep and allow your breath to relax you more and more. When you breathe in it energizes the body while the outgoing breath brings relaxation. Now drop all sense of urgency or any need to attend to anything else. Just be aware of your body and the breath. Surrender the whole body to the floor and let go. Make sure you don't fall asleep.

Step-7: After 10-20minutes when you feel fully relaxed keep your eyes closed and slowly roll onto your right side. Be in that position for approx a minute. Then, taking the support of your right hand, slowly sit up into a seated pose such as easy Pose (Sukhasana).

Step-8: Now keep your eyes closed and take a few deep breaths in and out as you gradually become aware of your environment and the body.

Step-9: After some time when you feel complete, slowly open your eyes.

Other benefits:

1. This yoga pose brings a deep, meditative state of rest, which helps in the

repair of tissues and cells, and in releasing stress. It also gives time for the yoga workout to sink in at a deeper level.

2. This pose leaves you in a state of rejuvenation. It is the perfect way to end a yoga session, particularly if it has been a fast-paced one.

3) Downward Facing Dog Pose (Adho Mukha Svanasana)

Instructions to perform this pose:

Step-1: First come onto your fours. Form a table such that your back forms the table top and your hands and feet form the legs of the table.

Step-2: While breathing out lift the hips up, straightening the knees and elbows, form an inverted V-shape with the body.

Step-3: Your hands should be shoulder width apart, feet should be hip width apart and parallel to each other. Toes point straight ahead.

Step-4: Now press your hands into the ground. Widen through the shoulder blades. Keep the neck lengthened by touching the ears to the inner arms.

Step-5: Now maintain this downward dog pose and take long deep breaths. Look towards the navel.

Step-6: While exhaling bend the knees, return to table pose. Relax.

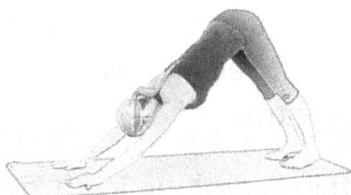

Fig. 2.3 Downward Facing Dog Pose

Precautions:

1. If you suffering from high blood pressure, detached eye retina, shoulder injury or diarrhoea then avoid this pose.

Other benefits:

1. This pose increases circulation of blood to the brain.

2. This pose is best way to calms the mind and helps relive headache, insomnia and fatigue.

4) Fish Pose

Instructions to perform this pose:

Step-1: First lie on your back. Your feet are together and hands relaxed alongside the body.

Step-2: Now place the hands underneath the hips, palms facing down and bring the elbows closer toward each other.

Step-3: While breathing in lift the chest up and head.

Step-4: Keep the chest elevated, lower the head backward and touch the top of the head to the floor.

Step-5: Press the elbows firmly into the ground, placing the weight on the elbow and not on the head with the head lightly touching the floor, Lift your chest up from in-between the shoulder blades. Now press the thighs and legs to the floor.

Step-6: Now maintain the pose for as long as you can with comfort and take gentle long breaths in and out. Relax in the posture with every exhalation.

Step-7: Now lift the head up, lowering the chest and head to the floor. Bring the hands back along the sides of the body and relax.

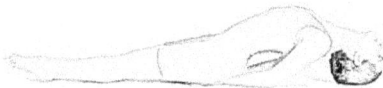

Fig. 2.4 Fish Pose

Precautions:

1. Avoid this pose if you have had serious lower-back or neck injuries .

2. Avoid this pose if you have high or low blood pressure.

Other benefits:

1. This pose helps relieve tension in the shoulders and neck.

2. This pose encourages deep breathing which helps in relief from respiratory disorders.

5) Head to Knee Pose

Instructions to perform this pose:

Step-1: First sit in Easy pose and extend the right leg straight out in front of you, place the bottom of the left foot against the right thigh. Pull the right leg in to square the hips to the front wall.

Step-2: While inhaling move the arms up and reach out of the waist lengthening the spine.

Step-3: Keep the length as you exhales forward, bending the right knee enough to interlace the fingers around the foot and to place the head against the knee.

Step-4: Press the head down into the knee to work the posture by, sliding the right heel away from you, lengthening the right leg. Maintain the head pressed to the knee while straightening the leg as much as you can. Press the heel away and pull the toes towards your head for a deeper stretch in the leg.

Step-5: Relax the shoulders and neck. Your shoulders should be parallel to the floor. Use the arms only enough to keep the head in contact with the knee.

Step-6: Breathe and hold for 3-6 breaths.

Step-7: When you release to the initial position inhale the arms up over your head, exhale them to the floor.

Step-8: Repeat the steps for other side.

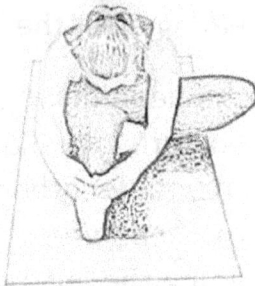

Fig. 2.5 Head to Knee Pose

Precautions:

1. Those who have recent or chronic back or knee injury should avoid this pose.

Other benefits:

1. This yoga pose calms the mind and emotions and helps stimulating the nervous, reproductive, endocrine and urinary systems.

6) Standing Forward Bend Pose

Instructions to perform this pose:

Step-1: First stand straight with feet together and arms alongside the body.

Step-2: You need to balance your weight equally on both feet.

Step-3: While breathing in extend your arms overhead.

Step-4: While breathing out bend forward and down towards the feet.

Step-5: Maintain this pose for 20-30 seconds and continue to breathe deeply.

Step-6: Keep the legs and spine erect; your hands rest either on the floor, beside the feet or on the legs.

Step-7: While you breathe out, move the chest towards the knees; lift the hips and tailbone higher; press the heels down; let the head relax and move it gently towards the feet. Keep breathing smoothly.

Step-8: While breathing in stretch your arms forward and up, slowly come up to the standing position.

Step-9: When you breathing out bring the arms to the sides.

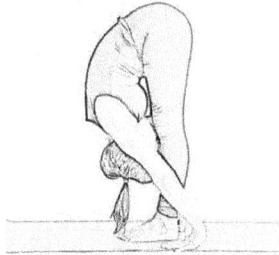

Fig. 2.6 Standing Forward Bend Pose

Precautions:

1. If you have back injury or any kind of spinal problems then you should not do this pose.

Other benefits:

1. This pose invigorates the nervous system by increasing the blood supply.

2. This pose makes the spine supple.

7) Legs Up The Wall Pose

Instructions to perform this pose:

Step-1: First lie down with your buttocks at the wall.

Step-2: Now try to extend your legs up the wall flex your toes towards you.

Step-3: Straight your knees by extending the hamstring.

Step-4: Now widen your legs slowly. Don't overstretch your thigh muscles.

Step-5: Keep flexing your feet toward you and try to keep your legs straight. You can use your hands if required.

Step-6: After few seconds come back to initial state. Relax.

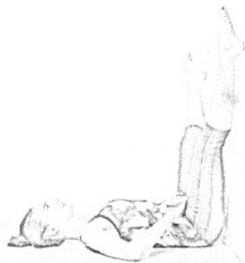

Fig. 2.7 Legs-Up-The-Wall Pose

Other benefits:

1. This is the best pose for stretching you thigh muscles.

8) Supported Chest Opener pose

Instructions to perform this pose:

Step-1: You should have blanket or thick towel.

Step-2: Now roll up the blanket or the towel you have.

Step-3: Lie down with the roll placed under your head.

Step-4: If necessary you can put pillow under your head.

Step-5: Close your eyes and relax. Stay in this position as long you like.

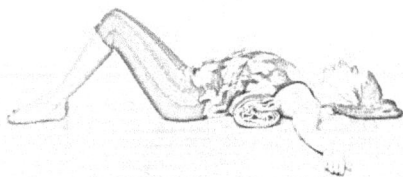

Fig. 2.8 Supported-Chest-Opener Pose

Other benefits:

1. This pose is mostly recommended after doing all other poses , it will help you in relaxing your body and gives great energy.

9) Child's Pose (Shishuasana)

Instructions to practice this pose:

Step-1: **First step is to s**it on your heels. Keep your hips on the heels and bend forward, after that lowers your forehead to the floor.

Step-2: Now Keep the arms alongside your body with hands on the floor, palms facing up. For beginners if this is not comfortable then you can place one fist on top of another and rest your forehead on them.

Step-3: Press your chest on the thighs gently.

Step-4: Hold this pose for few seconds.

Step-5: Slowly come up on the heels and sit cross leg(lotus position) and relax.

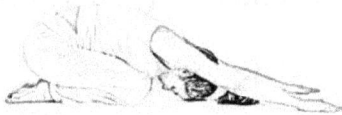

Fig. 2.9 Child's Pose

Precautions:

1. Pregnant women should avoid practicing this pose.

2. If you have suffered from diarrhoea recently then avoid this pose.

Other benefits:

1. This pose helps relieve constipation.

2. Child pose deeply relaxes your back.

10) Tree Pose (Vrikasana)

Instructions to practice this pose:

Step-1: First step is to stand straight with arms by the side of your body. Now bend your right knee and place the right foot high up on your left thigh. The sole of the foot should be placed flat and firmly near the root of the thigh.

Step-2: Your left leg should be straight. Maintain the balance of your body.

Step-3: Once you feel balanced then slowly raise your arms over your head from the side, and bring your palms together in hands-folded position (Namaste mudra).

Step-4: Now look straight ahead in front of you. A steady gaze would help to maintain a steady balance.

Step-5: Your spine should be straight and your entire body should be taut, like a stretched elastic band.

Step-6: Maintain deep breath and just be with your body and have a gentle smile on your face.

Step-7: Now exhale slowly and bring down your hands from sides. Gently release your right leg.

Step-8: Now you are in initial position. Repeat this pose with left leg off the ground on the right thigh.

Step-9: Relax.

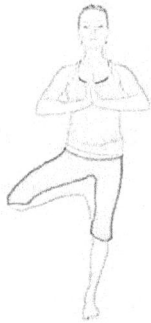

Fig. 2.10 Tree Pose

Precautions:

1. If you are suffering from migraine, insomnia, low or high blood pressure then avoid practicing this pose.

Other benefits:

1. This pose helps improve concentration.

2. This pose leaves you in state of rejuvenation and brings balance and equilibrium to your mind.

Chapter 19: Tips In Finding Inner Peace

Silence your thoughts.

When you feel like you're being overwhelmed by your thoughts, try to put on a mental break. Consciously put a stop to the swirling ideas in your head and start breathing. Breathe in and out. Thing of one object or a person and focus your thoughts and attention into it or him in order to calm your mind.

Know that things will pass.

The saying, "The only thing that is constant is change" may be one of the most overused and cliché lines ever but it does us some good to realize how true it is. Whatever problems you may have right now will pass. Your life can and will change for the better. Keep patient and let things happen naturally. If you don't believe that you will overcome your situation, you will get stuck and can't move on.

Finish what you start.

If you started something, end it. Don't leave it hanging. Closure is one of the keys for a tranquil and peaceful mind. No matter what business it is, it will do you good to follow through. Do you have a friend you haven't forgiven? Forgive him and save yourself the sleepless nights and the stress from the strained relationship. How about projects you've started but have never finished? You know what to do. Whether you're aware of it or not, unfinished business will actually weigh heavily on your mind and will bite you in the ass in the future.

Don't worry too much.

As much as you can, stop getting anxious even over the smallest of things. And don't waste all your time thinking about what **might** happen because this will surely create unnecessary turmoil and dread in your mind. **I might be late. I might not have enough money for groceries. There might be a problem with the work I submitted. I might fail**. Do you know what you need to focus on? Concentrate on the things you want, not on what you don't.

Live in the present.

Don't dwell in the past. You can't change it but you can learn something from it. Spend just enough time to think of what lessons you can take from what happened before to be better but never use the past as an escape. Pay attention to the present and don't let life pass you by.

Work on a single task.

Avoid multitasking. The quality of your work will suffer that way. Focus on a single task and do it well. Juggling things all at once will require a great amount of energy that will fatigue both your mind and body.

Don't procrastinate.

Procrastination seems to be the fad, nowadays. But what people don't realize is how procrastination is not beneficial to one's mental state. It just prolongs the tension and stress associated with a certain activity. It also adds additional pressure when you feel like you can't accomplish your tasks anymore because you've procrastinated way too long.

Usually, the things that we delay accomplishing are tedious, difficult, and uninteresting tasks like homework, paying the bills, and doing household chores, among others.

Learn how to say no.

Especially if you're the kind of person who treasures relationships and bonds so much to the point of not doing anything that might upset that connection, don't live your life by continually saying "yes" even when the answer should be "no."

Learn to speak up and refuse if you can't do something a person is asking of you. Learn that there will be times when you have to think of yourself and stop trying to please everyone. Learn to say no to what you know will stress you out.

Educate yourself.

Knowledge is power and being aware would make you feel more in control of yourself, your actions, and your thoughts. When you know you possess the necessary information, you will feel more confident and calm when it comes to everyday dealings. Sometimes, the reason why our minds aren't settling down is it's trying to solve a problem that we are not equipped enough to solve. If this is the case, then take the initiative to arm yourself with knowledge so you don't go into life half-blind.

And I'm not just talking about book knowledge, about knowing what one plus one is. Know why people act the way they do. Know what must be done in specific situations. Know the realities behind social conventions. Know if there's an alternative way to living.

Love yourself the way you want to be loved by others.

We love the iPod. We love the new ice cream shop just right around the corner. We love a lot of things but what we fail to love the most is ourselves. We place too much hate, pressure, blame, and insecurities on ourselves and at times, we even want to get out of our skin. All those stuff running around your head, your self-doubts and self-incriminations, are results of a lack of appreciation for the being that you are. Only when we are comfortable with the person that we are do we start to live a more stable, fulfilling, and worry-free life.

Focus on the positive.

There are two sides to a coin. For every bad thing that happens, there's always sometime positive that you can get out of the experience. Let's say you lost your wallet. Instead of moaning over the loss, think about how a person who is badly in need of finances could have found it and used it to solve some problem. Think about how that incident could teach you to be more careful next time.

Keep a gratitude list.

This not only paves the way for a peaceful mind but also for a happier one. Every day, make a list of three, five, or ten things that you are grateful for. Or list the events that made you happy. This way, you will end your day with a lighter mood and you will achieve an attitude that's optimistic about what the future have in store for you.

Understand your principles and values.

Whenever a crisis arises, there are times when we get conflicted as to how to respond. Somebody asks for our stand regarding a certain issue and we butt our heads against the wall trying to decide on the matter. What you need to do is understand and remember what you believe in, your principles, and your values. Always keep them in mind and let these life principles guide you. This way, whenever you're faced with a challenge, you know that you possess certain values that can battle the problem. Whenever something shakes your faith about what you believed in, just remember to stick to your principles to have a clearer and untroubled mind.

Learn to surrender.

We have to accept that we have no way of predicting every outcome. Sometimes, sad as it may sound, we don't have the answers and we can't control all situations. So surrender. Don't continuously fight against the tide. Let your life unfold as it may and don't get upset over the fact that things are taking you towards paths you've never imagined you'll be traveling in.

Don't wallow in sadness.

Find something to smile about. Don't dwell on the sad things that just happened to you. Negative emotions are a given in life but if you want to have a more serene state of mind, don't let them run the show. Sometimes, things just don't go the way we plan them to but staying miserable about it won't take away the pain.

Know that you are not alone.

You're going through some financial difficulties. You just broke up with the person you love. You're not quite sure if you'll still have a job tomorrow. And worse, you feel all alone amidst all the struggles you're experiencing. But you're wrong. Someone could be wearing the exact same shoes you have on. Don't ever think that you're the only person out there who's in misery. Take comfort from the thought that others have went through all your troubles and survived. If you can, seek these people out and ask for some advice, ask them what they did to get through the storm.

Don't let expectations rule your life.

We always have an ideal state of things, ideal way of life, ideal set of clothes and expected salary and desired place of living. We expect to raise this certain amount of money by the following year. It's perfectly okay to set aims for yourself and look at these expectations as end goals. But living only for the sake of fulfilling them will not bring you any peace of mind. They will rule your life instead of you ruling them. Furthermore, they will create unnecessary pressure that could make you intensely apprehensive and unsettled.

Meditate.

One of the prevailing methods that people use nowadays to find inner peace of mind is meditation. It's a very effective relaxation technique that you can do to reach a state of stillness without your mind and body. Doing meditation at least

once a week can lead you to achieve the
inner peace that you greatly need.

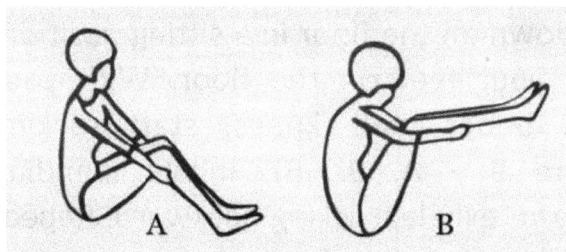

Chapter 20: Posture Exercises

7. Rocking Exercises

Get down on the floor in a sitting position; keep your feet on the floor. With your hand under your knees, start rocking (Figure 9 – A, 9 –B). Inhale, bending forward; exhale, rocking backward. Repeat ten times. Relax for a moment. This exercise is excellent for limbering up.

Figure 9 - Rocking Exercises

8. Gas-Relieving Posture

a. Lie flat on your back. Inhale, drawing up each knee alternately, pulling your knee onto your chest with both hands (Figure 10 – A). Holding the breath, stretch the leg (Figure 10 –B); then, exhaling return to starting position. Repeat twice.

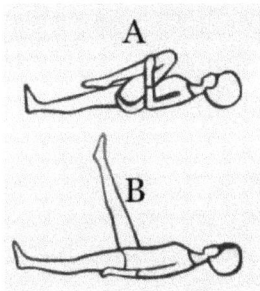

Figure 10 - Gas-Relieving Posture (A,B)

b. Inhale, drawing up both knees (Figure 11 – C). Holding the breath, stretch your legs up (Figure 11 –D); then, exhaling, slowly bring them down to starting position. Repeat twice. The principal muscles at work here are the upper and lower abdominals.

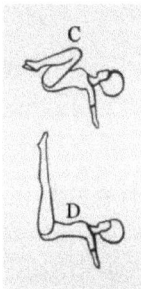

Figure 11 - Gas-Relieving Posture (C, D)

9. Leg Exercises

a. Lie flat on your back, hands along your sides. Inhale, raising the right leg (Figure 12 – A). Hold your breath for a moment. Exhale while slowly bringing the leg down. Repeat the same with your other leg, then with both legs at the same time (Figure 12 –B). It takes practice to bring both legs down slowly, so perform it gradually; do not force it. Women with female disorders should consult their doctor before practicing this pose.

b. Lie flat, arms above your head (Figure 12 – C). Now turn your whole body to the right, resting your head on your arm (Figure 12- D). Inhale, lifting your leg as high as you can (Figure 12 – E). Exhale, bringing your leg to the starting position. Repeat three times with each leg.

c. Still flat on the floor, inhale, lifting your leg as high as you can. Holding your breath, bring your leg down to the floor sideways (Figure 12 – F). Exhale and bring your leg to the starting position. Repeat twice with each leg. This posture strengthens abdominal muscles and reduces fat.

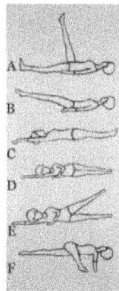

Figure 12 - Leg Exercises

10. The Arched-Back Posture

Lie flat on your back. Pull up your feet along the floor, a close to the body as you can, knees and heels together (Figure 13 – A), arms out slightly to the side. Inhale; raise the body, holding your breath (Figure 13 – B). Exhale, lowering your body to the floor. Repeat three times. This posture strengthens the back.

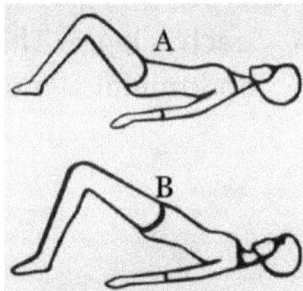

Figure 13 - The Arched-Back Posture

11. The Reverse or Plough Posture and the Shoulder-stand

a. Flat on your back, raise your legs, supporting the body with the hands. Close your eyes and do the deep breathing, inhaling and exhaling. Remain in this posture for 30 seconds and increase to 60 seconds (Figure 14- A).

b. From this posture, slowly lower both legs over your head, as far as you can go, but do not force it (figure 14 –B). Inhale while you are doing it. Now slowly start coming down, vertebra by vertebra. Exhale, and continue inhaling and exhaling as you bring your feet down. This exercise keeps your spine flexible and youthful. Repeat twice.

c. To do the shoulder-stand, use the same technique as in above; the body, however, should be in an absolutely straight position (Figure 14 – C). Practice the shoulder-stand only after you have made progress and feel that you can do the more difficult postures. When you are finished, rest your body flat on your back.

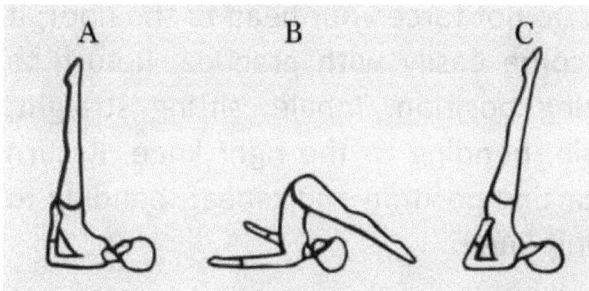

Figure 14 - The Reverse/Plough Posture

12. The Lotus Posture

a. This posture is the symbol of yoga and is used during meditation. Sit straight; cross your legs, placing the heel on the opposite thigh (Figure 15 -A). This pose is difficult and requires practice. Do not force yourself. Practice for the Lotus Posture as follows:

1. Sit tailor fashion (Figure 15 –B) until your muscles and joints are supple enough to feel comfortable in the Lotus position.

2. Still sitting tailor fashion, spine straight, inhale with your hands clasped behind your back. Exhale, bending down until your forehead touches the floor (Figure 15 – C). Do not force your head to the floor; it will come easily with practice. Return to starting position. Inhale, sitting straight; exhale, bending to the right knee. Return to starting position and repeat, bending to the left knee.

3. Another way to practice the Lotus Posture is: In a sitting position, place your foot on the opposite thigh and bounce the

knee until it touches the floor (Figure 15 – D). Repeat with the other foot.

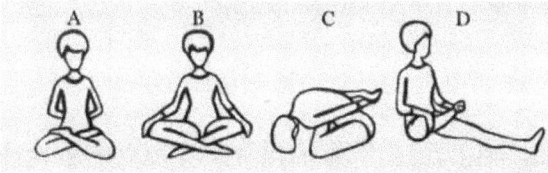

Figure 15 - The Lotus Posture

4. Sit straight. Inhale, legs stretched out, feet together. Exhale, bending down, hands stretched out until they reach your feet. In the beginning, it may be difficult to get your head as far down as your knees.

5. Return to sitting position. Inhale, legs apart. Exhale, bending forward, hands reaching your toes, head as low as possible. Return to starting position. Repeat three times.

6. Do the same as above, bending your head first to one knee, then to the other. Now relax, stretching flat on the floor for at least 60 seconds.

13. Neck Exercises

Sit tailor-fashion on the floor, spine straight, completely relaxed.

a. Throw the head back, then forward.

b. Turn the head to the right with a jerk, then to the left with a jerk.

c. Tilt the head sideways to the right, ear to shoulder. Repeat on the left side.

d. Rotate the head clockwise and counterclockwise, letting it relax completely, not forcing the motion.

These exercises are excellent for releasing tension around the neck. Repeat each exercise ten times. Finish by patting the neck and back with your hands. These exercises can be done at any time; they don't have to be included during your morning practice. If you are subject to dizziness, seek the services of your doctor before doing any of the postures, especially the neck exercises.

14. Eye Exercises

Again sit tailor-fashion on the floor, spine straight and completely relaxed.

a. Look up at the ceiling, then down at the floor. Blink and close your eyes lightly.

b. Move your eyes to the right, then to the left, without moving your head. Blink and close your eyes lightly.

c. Move your eyes up to the right, then down to the left. Blink and close your eyes lightly. Repeat, looking up to the left first, then down to the right.

d. Roll both eyes clockwise and counterclockwise.

e. Now shift the eyes: Choose an object close to the eyes, then shift them to an object in the far distance. Blink and close your eyes lightly.

Repeat each eye exercises from six to ten times, keeping the head straight, moving only the eyes.

15. Palming

Cover your eyes with your cupped hands. Rest the heels of your palms on your cheekbones without pressing them, fingers crossed over your forehead. Close your eyes lightly. The head should not be bent forward, but kept straight, without any strain on your nerves or muscles. Try to see black. Place your elbows on a pillow to elevate your position. Palming relieves common eyestrain and is helpful for people who do a great deal of reading or figure work. Palm for about two or three minutes at a time.

The eye exercises and palming can also be done during the day in case you have to rush through the morning practice session.

16. The Twist

Sitting on the floor, legs stretched out in front of you (Figure 16 –A). Slowly bend your left foot and place it under your right thigh. Then pull up your right leg and position it diagonally over your bent left leg, your right toes pointing outward (Figure 16 - B). Now grasp your right toe with your left hand, your right hand placed in the back at your waistline (Figure 16 – C). Inhaling a deep breath, get into the position and, while exhaling, slowing start twisting your head, shoulder, and waist to the right, as far as you can. Do not force it; the skill will come with practice. Repeat three times. Change the position of your legs and hands and repeat the exercise, facing the other direction.

Conclusion

Thank you again for downloading this book!

I hope this book was able to help you to understand what yoga is and how you can benefit from the practice, especially when it comes to mudras and asanas.

The next step is to practice what you have learned and make yoga as part of your everyday routine in order to alleviate stress and enjoy an everlasting physical and emotional health.

Thank you and good luck!

www.ingramcontent.com/pod-product-compliance
Lightning Source LLC
Chambersburg PA
CBHW051723020426
42333CB00014B/1123